The Power of Disruption

The Power of Disruption

A Memoir of Discovery

Susan Cross

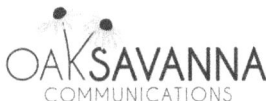

OAKSAVANNA
COMMUNICATIONS

Published by Oak Savanna Communications

ISBN: 978-1-7335584-1-9 (paperback)
ISBN: 978-1-7335584-0-2 (e-book)

Book design by: Christy Collins, Constellation Book Services
Cover photo by: Jon Cross
Author photo by: Mary Pencheff, Mary Pencheff Photography
For more information, visit susan-cross.com
Printed in the United States of America

Publisher's Cataloging-in-Publication Data

Names: Cross, Susan S., author.
Title: The Power of disruption : a memoir of discovery / Susan Cross.
Description: Whitehouse, OH: Oak Savanna Communications, 2019.
Identifiers: LCCN | ISBN 978-1-7335584-1-9 (pbk.) | 978-1-7335584-0-2 (e-book)
Subjects: LCSH Cross, Susan. | Spiritual biography. | Near-death experiences--Biography. | Rehabilitation. | Self-actualization (Psychology). | Healing. | Conduct of life. | BISAC BODY, MIND & SPIRIT / Healing / Prayer & Spiritual | BODY, MIND & SPIRIT / Parapsychology / Near-Death Experience | BIOGRAPHY & AUTOBIOGRAPHY / Personal Memoirs | SELF-HELP / Motivational & Inspirational.
Classification: LCC BF575.H27 .C76 2019 | DDC 158/.1/0924--dc23

Library of Congress Control Number: 2019900353

For Jon
the love of my life and my best friend

Author's Note

This book is a memoir, and it is drawn from my own experience. All the names of the people we met in Dominica have been changed or disguised to afford them their privacy. The exception is Hervé Nizard, our host at Citrus Creek Plantation, who kindly granted me permission to use his real name. The names of my family members are real and used with permission. Names of specific locations are real.

Contents

Introduction

On January 30, 2017, my life changed forever. That was the day that I "died." I don't know for how long, and I can't say that my heart stopped beating, I took a dramatic last breath, or any of the usual changes that can happen to a physical body when it ceases to be part of this earthly plain. But something happened that forced my life to come to a screeching halt in more ways than one. That was the day that I left this earth and transcended into another space and, quite literally, time stopped.

Obviously, I'm still here, so I didn't die by the usual definition. Let's call it a traumatic, dramatic pause that changed me forever immediately and in ways that I'm still discovering. It forced me to look closer at who I am, what I stand for, and what my purpose really is. It's when life got both harder and simpler at the same time.

The timing of my death was unexpected, yet the fact that it happened really wasn't. Looking back on it, I think it had been building for some time—maybe even my whole life. In that moment and all the moments since, it was as real to me as the words on this page. In fact, it's hard to truly describe how real it was—and still is.

What happened? The medical answer is that my appendix ruptured while on vacation on the remote Caribbean island of Dominica and my body filled with infection. I almost died. The emotional answer is that I had to surrender fully to the circumstances of my emergency surgery and recovery to restart my life. The spiritual answer is that in the midst of the poison of sickness and pain, I felt myself leave my earthly life to be bathed in light—a warm light so bright and full of hope, safety, comfort, promise, and joy that I wanted more and more of it. In short, I was reminded unequivocally that I matter, and my eyes opened to the mission all of us should be pursuing: living our best authentic life possible.

I have a gnawing need in my heart to share my story. Even when I was going through everything, I took notes on my phone because there was so much happening I knew I'd need to be able to process it all at a later time. I tried to fight writing the memoir and delayed starting anything in earnest until I hit the six-month anniversary of my surgery. That milestone, followed closely by an opportunity to hear firsthand the story of a survivor of the 2013 Boston Marathon bombing, made me change the way I think about the reactions of most who hear my story. I went through something scary, bold, amazing, and life changing. It meant something to me and maybe it can provide some inspiration for others, too.

Wishing you love and peace,

Susan

A Life Spinning
Out of Control

The first time I remember being told I had to change the way I thought so I could fit in was in kindergarten. I could already read, and my teacher made us practice some phonics lessons and then color the worksheets. I was bored and colored each of the nine images on the page purple. My teacher sent a note to my parents and the next day, my dad went in for a conference because my mom was home with a toddler and my baby brother.

Since I wasn't a kid who usually got into trouble at school, I had no idea what was going on. When my dad got home, he and my mom weren't mad, but they told me very clearly that there would be times in life when I'd have to follow all the rules given to me by people in authority in order to get along. Coloring correctly on phonics papers fell into this category.

Despite this early lesson, my parents and others encouraged me to develop my whole self and gave me a lot of freedom to learn new things as I grew up. I grew confident in my own voice, and in my right to have one, but I also heard a consistent message of caution when it came to showing the world my true self.

Fast forward to adulthood. The messages of my youth convinced me I wasn't good enough as me. Me being me could be a disruption to those around me. I had to conform to the standards others were able to tolerate in order to be recognized, appreciated, and valued, even if they were asking to know my true thoughts. So, I worked hard to adapt and thought I had to be an overachiever to find my space in the world.

My resumé as a public relations professional and marketing communications strategist has been hard-earned. I'm generally known as a high performer and team leader with a reputation for delivering results. Over time, my unique way of thinking earned praise and recognition because of what it could do for others. "At last," I told myself, "I have value!" Lucky me! Well, not really. I mistakenly believed that my self-worth was attached to what others told me I did well because it was important to them. I wasn't sure who I was if I wasn't fulfilling a specific role. I didn't know how to just be me.

While I had been living the American dream of success on paper, my world was rapidly becoming a series of compartmentalized experiences rather than one authentic life. On the outside I gave the appearance of focus and presence. On the inside, I was often miles away. Did I like what I was doing? You bet. It's amazing to stretch the brain, achieve professional success, and get paid for telling stories. Did I like myself while I was doing this? Not always. I just didn't realize it.

All I knew was that I was getting tired. My car knew its own way to the airport. I was fitting in time with my husband and kids. I was gaining weight and not making as much time as usual for exercise. I was receiving all the outward accolades of a life well lived, while on the inside I was slowly losing a connection to myself. Did I really know what was most important any longer? No. The truth is that I was living a life designed for future approvals without fully embracing the good of each moment *now*.

By the end of 2016, it had been nearly two years since I'd taken a real vacation, one that didn't require me to check in daily or set aside one to two hours per day to keep projects moving through the boutique advertising agency where I worked. I'd been traveling a lot but was looking forward to visiting the remote Caribbean island of Dominica, known for its hiking and snorkeling, with my husband, Jon. Our late-January travel dates would be a nice respite from the hectic agency pace that had become normal. And they were just ahead of another busy, multiweek travel season for me.

This vacation was important, and I was ready to enjoy the sunshine, pristine waters, and slower pace that are uniquely Caribbean.

Choosing Dominica

My husband, Jon, and I are active vacationers. We hike, bike, kayak, and explore. Our main goal for every vacation is to just *be* and we usually don't overschedule. Our usual lives and jobs are highly structured, and we're generally surrounded by people. We've enjoyed the work and it's provided our family with a very nice life. When you're used to such a fast pace, vacation time is down time to shut off the brain and reconnect mind, body, and spirit.

This had long been the case, but once our kids left home for college and life pursuits of their own, we started treating ourselves to more frequent trips and getaways to remote locations. We like to rent a house or cabin and hit the grocery and farm stand to stock up on local food and drink. This allows us to set our own schedule and keeps our supplies fresh for day trips. We often visit local bars and restaurants, but after a long day's trek, we love coming back to our rented home base to relax.

During a hike on St. John in the US Virgin Islands one year, we met a retired couple who were talking about the wonders of Dominica, known as "the nature island" due to its spectacular flora and fauna, much of which is protected by an extensive national park system. Eco-tourism is popular on the island and it's also a popular honeymoon spot and cruise ship day trip. We were intrigued and told ourselves that we'd visit one day. That day finally came in January 2017.

The unique combination of rugged, natural beauty and all the comforts of home grabbed our attention. Jon was enjoying a work sabbatical and researched and booked everything for the trip. He found a wonderful cottage to rent on a working tropical fruits plantation located on the east coast of the island. This side of the island is known for being quieter and the landscape wilder than the west side, where all the cruise ships stop and where the main city of Roseau is located.

Citrus Creek Plantation is located on twenty acres along the banks of the Taberi River near the small town of La Plaine. There are twelve rental cottages and villas plus a restaurant. It's owned and operated by Hervé "RV" Nizard and that comforted us. While we are well traveled, we felt that it was important to stay somewhere that a local could help us if necessary. How fortunate that decision turned out to be.

All accommodations at the resort are open-air Caribbean style, combining the best of both outdoor living and the comforts of home. We chose the Banyan Stone Tree House, a seven-hundred-fifty-square-foot stone cottage built into the coconut ridge around a huge Banyan tree. It was very private and exclusive, which gave us the feeling of being alone in the jungle with earthy smells and the soothing natural music of bird, ocean, and insect sounds. The fully equipped kitchen was located outside on the lanai with a gorgeous view of the sea, mountains, and plantation. The bathroom was inside, but for extra fun, the shower was located outside in the roots of the Banyan tree! We were all set for another new experience, one we could never find back in the States.

An Island Paradise

Dominica is not easy to get to. It's about halfway between the French islands of Guadeloupe to the north and Martinique to the south. The island is small at only about 290 square miles but is still the fourth largest island in the eastern Caribbean. Many people have never heard of this island nation and frequently confuse it with the Dominican Republic. A mere 29.2 miles long and 18 miles wide, Dominica faces the Atlantic Ocean to the east and the Caribbean Sea to the west. More than seventy thousand people live there, and most of the residents are of African or Carib descent. About fifteen thousand residents live in the capital of Roseau, which is on the southwest coast.

Dominica—called Waitikubuli, or "Tall is her Body," by native Caribs—had been claimed by both the French and the British, but it has been independent since 1978. It is known for having one of the most rugged landscapes of the Caribbean and is covered by a largely unspoiled, multilayered rainforest. It is also among the earth's most rain-drenched lands, and the water runoff forms cascading rivers, waterfalls, and natural pools. Much of the island is protected as three national parks and multiple World UNESCO sites are found there. It's also known as a birder's paradise as it is home to some species that are considered endangered or extinct on other Caribbean islands. Its highest peak, Morne Diablotins, is nearly five thousand feet. The country's central spine is a northwest-southeast axis of steep volcanic slopes and deep gorges. East-west mountain spurs extend to a narrow coastal plain, which is studded with sea cliffs. There are eight or nine active volcanoes on the island.

As we flew in, our view from the air was of this rugged landscape and no evidence of civilization. It was jungle—pure bush—completely covering jagged mountains. We could clearly see the sweeping landscape and the beautiful blues and greens of the Caribbean Sea and the Atlantic Ocean. It was breathtaking. All of a sudden, an airstrip came into view. One minute we were flying and the next we were literally cutting through the jungle toward a narrow runway leading toward a very small airport. The remoteness was just what we wanted.

We were eager to get to our rental after nearly a full day of travel. It was getting dark and Citrus Creek had a driver waiting for us. We travel light—one suitcase and one backpack each—and squeezed into a small compact car with our driver and another man who appeared to be a driver-in-training. Our driver, a preacher by day, welcomed us warmly.

Thank goodness we had a driver! We're pretty easygoing when it comes to embracing local culture and practices, but from the very first ride, we knew that travel here would be anything but ordinary.

First, Dominicans drive on the left side of the road, a nod to the era in which they were under British rule. Second, to reach our final destination, we had to travel ten to twelve miles across the island, which takes about one hour over a winding, mountain road that is about one and half lanes wide. In most places, there were no guardrails, and in many places, the road was washed out, damaged, full of potholes, or being repaired. Third, there were no lights on most of the road except for the car's headlights. And to add another degree of difficulty, the car was American-style with the steering wheel on the left side.

When we arrived, we were greeted by Citrus Creek's owner, Hervé, who invited us to dine at the restaurant. We eagerly accepted and enjoyed a delicious meal. Our first introduction to Citrus Creek and our vacation was just what we'd hoped for: good food, nice people, natural surroundings, and quiet. Hervé drove us in our rental car to the Banyan Stone Cottage, where we showered and slept soundly in our jungle paradise.

On our first full day, Tuesday, I got up, fixed myself some mint herbal tea, and sat on the lanai to email the kids that we'd arrived safely. The cottage had WiFi, which we used to keep in touch with the kids, but otherwise we enjoyed being cut off from our normal lives for the most part. Although I had promised myself (and Jon) I wasn't going to work, I had a lot going on that wasn't able to be completed before our trip and had agreed to check email once a day. Jon supported this and I limited my checking in to mornings for about an hour or so. After that, I'd read one of the many books on my iPad while I waited for Jon to wake up.

While I was sitting there, taking it all in, a little bananaquit bird landed on the table next to me, the first of a few such visits. I noticed that he had only one foot, but that didn't stop him from bopping around. I kept my movements to a minimum so I wouldn't scare him away, but he didn't show any fear. In fact, it felt like he was staring at me and sizing me up somehow. He didn't chirp or sing, but I swear that he looked me directly in the eyes and connected with me as if he were saying, "Good morning! Enjoy the day! You've come to the right place!" I remember thinking that it was a miracle that he'd survived with only one foot. That had to make landings and perching to eat pretty challenging. It didn't seem to slow him down, though. In fact, I told the kids he might have had only one foot, but he was a good flier. After about five minutes or so, he flew off. I just sat there, read, and breathed. This was going to be an amazing vacation!

The best thing about vacation for me is the mind-set. It's the ultimate permission to simply stand down and live unscheduled. I'm a classic type-A personality—a real driver who is used to being on the go and multitasking. I go all in almost all the time, whether I'm at work or play. Most of my days are highly structured and deadline driven. I live by my calendar and usually recite it at least sixty days out.

On vacation, I'm the opposite. No makeup, hair under a hat, no clocks, minimal technology. My biggest decisions are what to eat and where to poke around to experience wherever I am. In fact, unless absolutely necessary, my husband and I don't even schedule anything except travel so we can absorb whatever we feel like being part of at any given moment.

When Jon finally got up, we discussed our plans for our first day. We agreed we wanted to get a better lay of the land near our cottage, and we started with a visit to the river and the nearby beach after having breakfast at the cottage. The river emptied into the ocean. We climbed around on the rocky beach beneath some cliffs. There's something so incredibly Zen-like for me when I'm around water. I can sit and stare out at the sea (or river or lake or pond) and just get lost in the beautiful rhythm of it. It's like my mind stops thinking through its usual checklist and becomes much more aware of the art of life and not the rigors of it. I can also tune out distracting sounds like cars, planes, and people and pay attention only to the sounds I want to hear, like birds and waves.

If you enjoy playing outside, then Dominica is the place to be. I've been lucky to travel all over the world and I've never seen a place with this kind of natural beauty. The jungle was lush and the water crystal clear. The mountains seemed to stand strong and proud as if they were watching over everything on the island. It's both quiet and noisy with the sounds of birds, insects, and water ever-present. What's missing are the sounds of civilization like technology, motors, and airplanes.

It was so nice to be with Jon without phone service or television to distract us from our rest and relaxation. When we travel, we always make sure that the kids can reach us either at the place where we're staying or via text on a special app that works when we're out of the United States (one of the perks of being married to an IT guy is that he's always on top of the latest and greatest technology!). We tell the rest of the family that if they need us, they can contact the kids, who can track us down. In over thirty years of travel together, we can count on one hand the number of times anyone has had an emergency and reached out. On day one of our trip, we had no clue that this time it would be us doing the reaching out.

Hiking, Touring, and Getting to Know Dominica

On Wednesday, we drove for an hour to travel eighteen miles across the island along a winding, narrow, pothole-strewn road to Champagne Beach, near the capital of Roseau. The beach isn't sandy. It's all rock, but beautiful in its own right. We had our own snorkel gear and, after stowing our shoes, entered the water to see the wonders below the surface.

A quick word about snorkeling and swimming . . . I'm a strong swimmer, but I'm also a floater. No matter what I do, my body wants to float. This makes it kind of hard for me to wear fins to snorkel. My legs want to rise to the surface of the water, which means I must work extra hard to use my fins to get anywhere. After a few minutes in the water at Champagne Beach, I realized that I'd need to wear my Tevas and ditch my fins, which I did. I dove in and joined Jon.

We've snorkeled in some beautiful places and this ranks as one of the best. The sun's rays broke through the surface of the water, casting beams of bright light down toward the rocks. Schools of colorful fish swam everywhere and darted in and out of the sunlight. One fish, a parrot fish, kept swimming by as if he were checking me out. I smiled through my mask because it reminded me of one of my daughter's favorite childhood books, *The Rainbow Fish*.

To top that off, champagne-like bubbles floated up to the surface from fissures in the volcanic rock (hence the name "Champagne Beach"). The bubbles come from a volcanic vent under the rocks in the water. Picture a glass of champagne and the subtle effervescence that allows the bubbles to gently rise to the top of the glass. Now, imagine that you're immersed in that glass and looking at the bubbles as they surround you. It's surreal to be in the midst of that.

Jon was off exploring in the water diving here and there, while many cruise ship tourists were snorkeling in guided groups. I swam close to one guide to hear what he was saying about the natural phenomena. Then, I stopped swimming and just laid on top of the water and let myself float. To be weightless in the water was so relaxing. I felt myself drifting as if I were being gently cradled in a hammock and rocked. It was so comforting and peaceful. I lazily watched the bubbles and the fish and listened to the quiet. Something about that place seemed to speak to my soul and remind me to appreciate the simple pleasures of nature—and I listened for once. I'm not sure how long I remained suspended on the water, but my prunelike fingertips told me that it was quite a while.

"Wasn't that amazing?" Jon said as we sat on the beach and removed our snorkeling gear. "I could hear the volcanic gases bubbling up through the fissures in the rock. Hey, are you okay?"

"I'm just tired," I said. "I think I'm still transitioning from work to vacation. Now that I'm relaxing, it's all catching up to me. I'll be fine."

"I'm hungry," Jon said. "I wonder what we'll find at the store."

"It's always an adventure to shop in the Caribbean," I laughed. "Fresh food is local and organic, but the variety is a little different than back home. I don't really have much of an appetite yet, but let's go."

We stowed our gear in our beach bags, dried off, and headed back to the car.

We stopped at a grocery store to stock up on the rest of our supplies and then made the long trek back to our cottage on the other side of the island.

The following day, Thursday, our third full day of the trip, we decided to find some hiking trails. Dominica is a hiker's paradise. There are hundreds of miles of trails that range from easy to treacherous. Its most famous trail, the renowned Waitikubuli National Trail, crosses the island. The first long-distance trail in the Caribbean, it's 115 miles long, has fourteen sections, and is rugged with no campsites. It's famous among hikers and people from all over the world come to hike this trail. We didn't hike the trail officially, but we did walk along a small part of it while visiting the Emerald Pool, a World Heritage Site located in Morne Trois Pitons National Park.

The Emerald Pool Trail was an easy manicured path to a waterfall falling into an emerald-colored pool of water. It was very pretty and is a popular stopping point for cruise ship travelers. Dominicans are very proud of this treasure and make sure it is well kept. Our leisurely walk was a lot of fun and a good start to the hiking part of our trip. I must admit that I was a little worried about seeing a snake on the trail. I'm afraid of snakes and know that while there aren't any poisonous snakes on Dominica, there are boa constrictors. Jon and I have a cardinal rule when we hike that he isn't allowed to point out any snakes he sees on the trail unless I'm in imminent danger of being bit. It's a rule that has stood us well on many a hike. We laugh about it, but in all these years, I can't think of one time he's broken it. I was praying that we didn't see any snakes. Luckily, we didn't.

When we got in the car to leave, a small tropical bird landed on the sideview mirror on my side of the car. It was the same kind of bird that had visited me at breakfast on our first morning on the island. It just sat there for a bit and looked at me as if it were checking me out. I mean, that bird really looked me in the eye.

It didn't flinch but studied me as if trying to connect with me in some way. I often have dogs, strangers, and children look at me as if they know me. They stare as if they're seeing right into my soul, as if they think I know something that they want to know or want to be part of me in some way. I had never paid much attention to it until Jon pointed it out. Anyway, this bird gave me that same look just as my breakfast companion did. It was weird, but not scary. After a short while it flew off. Both Jon and I smiled and commented that even the birds on Dominica were friendly!

From the Emerald Pool we went to go find a place called the Jacko Steps, which was billed as an easy hike by Dominican standards and had some history attached to it that intrigued us. This trail is named after a runaway slave named Jacko, who was the leader of a group of escaped slaves, known as Maroons, in the 1700s. The Maroons carved steps up the side of a mountain to the place where they lived for about one hundred years. The steep flight of 135 steps, each about two feet high, requires that you literally pull yourself up each one.

We arrived at where we thought the trail should be, then drove up and down the road a couple of times looking for the trailhead. Eventually we pulled over to look at the map some more. Not many places of interest are marked in Dominica. They're on maps but there are very few signs along the road to tell you where they are. We were still unsure even after checking the map, so we decided to get out of the car and ask for help. We approached an older local guy working on the road and he told us in the Caribbean English of Dominica that we just happened to be in the right place. He explained in detail how to get to the trail, but he was very hard to understand. I was at a loss. All Jon could understand was to walk down this gravel road and cross the river—the Layou River—which was in a beautiful gorge. According to Jon, "After that I was lost."

We headed back to the car to get our boots and other hiking gear. About that time a small dog ran under our car. He was an adorable mutt and full of energy with a tail that wouldn't stop wagging. Once we had our hiking boots on, the dog, who had been patiently waiting, took off down the paved road ahead of us. Jon heard the old man yell, "Follow the dog!" and he thought, "Great, now we're at the mercy of a dog as a trail guide."

We headed down the road for maybe seven hundred feet. The path was lined with gorgeous, bright red and pink flowers. We could hear the river in the distance. When we got to the river, the dog was there waiting for us. He really was our trail guide! The dog bounced across the rocks in the river and scrambled up the other side of the bank and waited. Clearly, we were supposed to follow. We took off our boots, but the river bottom was too rocky to walk across barefoot. Jon went back to the car to get our sandals while I waited on the riverbank. With sandals on, we made it across the shallow river and the dog, who had disappeared for a bit, was waiting for us once again. He acted like we were supposed to go one direction, but we went the other way until we realized it wasn't right. We turned back, found the trail, paid the local nature organization a small fee to walk it, and climbed up the hill to the top of the Jacko Steps.

We arrived at the top of the steps and would descend toward the river. Jon, of course, was a champion. (I think he's part mountain goat the way he attacks climbing!) I did well on the climb down, especially since climbing isn't one of my big strengths. Those steps were steep! I must admit that some of the time I sat down and butt-slid from step to step. Hey, don't laugh (even though Jon did—although after more than thirty years, I don't think anything about me surprises him anymore)! And, don't ever underestimate the value of a good butt slide when it comes to a steep descent!

Once we reached the riverbank, we considered our options: walk back down the river to the car or climb the 135 steps we had just descended and return to our starting point. The river was high and fast with what appeared to be whitecaps swirling every once in a while. The water was clean and clear, except where debris had been churned up from the fast flow. We'd passed a few hikers on the trail who had swum downriver and climbed up the steps. They were traversing the trail in the opposite direction than we were. They told us that their "float" was fun, but that it was also a little scary due to the strong current. We're good swimmers and usually up for a water adventure, but we weren't feeling it at that time. The current was pretty strong, and we didn't want to take any unnecessary risks. We decided to go back the same way we had come.

Jon, of course, skirted up the steps as if they were nothing. I was still gaining my balance and couldn't shake the mental exhaustion of being on such a fast work and life pace before vacation. To be honest, although I knew I had to climb my way out, I was dreading it. I wasn't just mentally tired, my body felt weighed down. When I reached the base of the steps, I looked up at the task before me, gave myself a good talking to, and started in. I was worried I might touch a snake or other critter as I clawed my way to the top by pretty much any means possible. All I kept thinking was that I was glad I was in good enough shape to make the hike and saying over and over, "One step at a time. One step at a time." It took me longer than Jon, but I did it! Once I got to the top, I was exhausted in every possible way, but also exhilarated.

On the drive back to our cottage, we stopped at another trail that was an easy walk back to a very nice waterfall. I was very tired, but Jon and I both figured it was due to the strenuous hike we just did. I wasn't especially sore or in pain, just zapped of energy. I was also starting to have some trouble concentrating, but I attributed that to the Jacko Steps hike. I was happy to let Jon be in charge and just be a follower for a bit. When we got back to our cottage, we enjoyed dinner on our lanai and just soaked in the sounds and smells of the jungle. It was a relaxing end to the day.

Jon told me later that when we got up Friday morning, I had a look on my face that he'd never seen in the thirty-plus years we've been together.

"Are you okay?" he asked. "You look like you're both mad and confused."

I could see a mix of genuine concern and compassion on his face, but I tried to make light of it.

"I'm fine," I replied. "I'm really tired. The hiking and snorkeling must have taken more out of me than I thought. Clearly, I didn't up my exercise game enough before we got here!"

I'd been pushing my body to help my mind relax and to restore my spirit, which all felt a little disconnected from each other. I didn't share this with Jon because I didn't think it was anything serious. Plus, I didn't want him to worry.

We stayed close to the cottage that day and walked along the beach across the road from our place. We then drove up the road to a trail that required climbing down a rope that hung over a tall cliff to the beach below. A waterfall in the cliff poured into the ocean. Jon did the climb down while I stayed at the trailhead. The trail looked amazing but hanging off a cliff on a rope isn't really my thing. Besides, I'd had a hard time with the small trail leading to the cliff and felt very tentative on it, and that was a well-manicured path. There were some steep spots, but it was really nothing that I couldn't have handled relatively well on a normal day.

My tentativeness was making me a little anxious, a feeling that I rarely have. It was as if my brain was starting to think at a faster pace than normal, kind of like when you speed up a video clip. Lacking another explanation, I attributed the feeling to coming down from an insane work schedule (average hours per week in the high fifties) and my body adjusting. There were no other incidents that day, but by the time I went to bed, I was bone tired.

On Saturday, we woke up refreshed, but I was still tired. We decided not to hike and went instead to a restored native village. It was located nearly all the way back to the airport—about an hour's drive across the island. It took some time to find the place, but once we did, the tour was wonderful and the enthusiasm and pride of the Dominicans working in the village made us feel like honored guests. We spent a couple of hours touring and learning the history of the native Caribs, then devoured a local dish with chicken, vegetables, and spices for lunch. It was delicious! Afterward, we drove the adventurous roads back to the cottage.

Our kids and their spouses had arranged for a private dinner to be prepared at our cottage that night. One of the chefs from the Citrus Creek restaurant and one of its general managers pulled out all the stops. Drinks, hors d'oeuvres, multiple courses—dinner was absolutely amazing! We were texting the kids photos and really enjoying ourselves. The seclusion of our cottage, the natural sounds, the great food—it was a fantastic cap to what had already been a great trip. There was just something about this place that seemed to be speaking to our souls.

Something's Not Right

The next morning, Sunday, I didn't feel well at all. I had lower abdominal and back pain and just felt generally bad. I told Jon to go ahead and do something on his own. I knew I needed to stay at the cottage that day and didn't want to stray too far from a Western-style bathroom. I could tell he was a little put out, but I could also tell that he needed some time alone. Jon drove a short way up the road to a spot where he wanted to hike. He spent a few hours walking a trail and looking out over a cliff across the ocean. He was back by about 2:00 p.m. and the photos looked amazing. It was definitely a place I wanted to see.

While he was gone, I'd spent some time on the lanai reading. After a bit, I couldn't concentrate anymore on the book. I was in pain but decided that a walk might make me feel better. I walked all around the Citrus Creek property and checked out some of the other cottages. I felt better at first just getting some exercise and I was able to make the steep climb down from our cottage easily. Then I started to hurt. I made it back to the cottage just in time to get violently sick from every possible orifice in my body. Since I'd had a local drink the night before that was served over ice before I realized it, in addition to the local lunch we'd eaten at the history center, I figured that I had a gastrointestinal issue going on that would run its course. Not fun, but nothing to worry about.

When Jon got back, he realized I'd gotten worse. I went to bed and Jon cooked himself something to eat.

Monday, January 30, became D-Day for us. I didn't sleep well all Sunday night and knew I needed another day of rest. Jon was slightly put out again by not being able to go see more of the island. I knew it and felt very guilty. This is one of the world's most beautiful and natural places, but we didn't have a chance to do everything on our bucket list. When Jon tells this part of the story, he admits that since it was the day before we were supposed to leave it made sense to make sure I was going to be okay. I still felt guilty, but at that point, I was getting so weak that I had to set aside worrying about him. I figured I'd apologize later and we'd work it out. Over the years, we've learned when to give and when to take.

I suspected a kidney stone and many of my symptoms went along with that theory. Thanks to the Internet, we tried to follow a home remedy for kidney stones of olive oil and lime juice followed by water and thirty minutes later another dose of lime juice with apple cider vinegar in water. Same thing an hour later. That didn't work. In fact, it resulted in vomiting a few times over the next hour or so. My body wasn't right, and it was telling me something. I just didn't know what. All I could think was that I needed to stabilize so that we could travel back to the United States as planned the next day. I was a little freaked out that if I appeared sick, I wouldn't get through Customs. There were some crazy restrictions being placed on travel in and out of the United States at that time and I didn't want us to get caught in the cross fire.

Jon got something to eat, cleaned up the cabin, and sat outside to read a book. I'd been dozing on and off but suddenly had uncontrollable shaking and chills and realized I had a fever. At that point, I got scared. Still believing I had a kidney stone, all I could think about was a friend I worked with in Michigan who had described the pain she felt when passing a kidney stone. Her description was vivid, gut-wrenching, and downright scary. I kept telling myself I could handle this. I mean, I'd had two babies naturally, for goodness' sake! This should be okay. I tried yoga breathing. I tried to focus my mind's eye on a warm fire in our fireplace at home. I piled on the covers. Nothing worked. My brain started to become a little foggy and I started to think I couldn't trust myself to get through this. I didn't want to worry Jon, but I knew I needed help. Now. I was freezing in the middle of a tropical paradise!

I half rolled, half fell out of bed and dragged myself to the lanai where Jon was reading. I asked him, through teeth chattering so hard that I thought I was going to crack one, if he could help me warm up. Although I thought I was calm when I talked to him, the look on his face said it all. He was scared for me and was going to do everything he could to help me feel better. He came in and lay down on the bed with me and tried to use his body heat to warm me up. Eventually, the convulsions stopped and I dozed again. I seemed temporarily stable, but in fact things had changed for the worse. Neither one of us knew just how much.

Jon talks about it this way: "In a minute, everything changed for me. I went down to speak with Hervé to see what our medical options were. He suggested the local health clinic in La Plaine, maybe a mile away. I felt like that was a move of desperation but at this point we were getting close to that. Susan couldn't stand up straight due to the pain, she couldn't keep anything inside of her, and she was having what seemed like convulsions. She was confused and said that she felt like she was watching all of this happen outside of her body."

Jon texted with our son, Jimmy, who was in the clinical portion of his training as a physician assistant at the time. Looking back on it, texting Jimmy was the right thing to do, but it put him in an awkward situation. He was clear that he couldn't diagnose me and that the texts weren't a substitute for on-site medical care. But he's a trained professional and our son. He wanted to help and was calm and professional when talking medicine. When I saw the texts later, I could tell he was worried. Jon described what was going on and Jimmy ran him through a list of questions to help assess my condition. He agreed that a trip to the clinic was the right choice.

Jon and I sat on the bed and talked about whether to go to the clinic. I was really starting to feel out of it. My body was barely holding itself together and my brain was so fogged that I was having trouble following our conversation. I had to force myself to stay as focused as possible and think through what to do next. It was as if I was submerged in water and trying to distinguish sounds but not really succeeding. I saw Jon's mouth moving and knew he was talking, but I was only catching part of his words.

As we were sitting there, I felt myself fade out mentally. I was on the edge of an empty, inky blackness that was trying hard to draw me in. In that moment, it would have been so easy to succumb to the nothingness. It seemed to offer me some relief from the pain and confusion I was feeling, but there was no sense of light, especially my light. No sense of healing other than pain relief. Something inside me told me to stay away from the blackness and to stay as alert as possible. I simply didn't want to surrender any part of myself. I felt like I needed to fight like heck to retain *me*.

It's a weird feeling to slowly lose control over your mind and body. It's scary but it's also surreal—like it's happening but also not happening. I felt like I was an amnesiac in a movie where life was happening around me, but I wasn't part of it and no one knew me. I realized on some level that I was on the verge of something I'd never experienced before. Sometimes it seemed like I was being pulled into a vast emptiness that I couldn't relate to. At the same time, I had this very strong sense that I didn't want to go there. It wasn't that the blackness itself was filled with terror; in fact, it seemed to promise a sense of calm. Somehow, I sensed that the calm would come at a price—a spiritual and mental void that I wasn't ready for.

Everything in me fought against going into the darkness. The closest I can come to describing it in real-life terms is that feeling you get when you're driving up a steep hill. The car is climbing steadily, but you can't see over the top of the peak. It's as if the world could end at the top. It's appealing to take the risk and part of you really wants to floor it over the top; but at the same time, it's frightening because of the unknown. I was worried about all this confusion going on in my brain, but I never thought I was closing in on life or death.

Jon helped me walk to the car and poured me in. I was barely able to stand up at that time without help and my abdomen and back were in excruciating pain. It wasn't like labor pains that come and go. It was more like one constant cramp that would not let up. Somewhere in my brain I remembered that it helped to apply reverse pressure for abdominal pain. I'd done that years ago while recovering from gall bladder surgery. It worked temporarily this time, but I still felt awful.

The Medical Adventure Begins

I've never had to receive medical care outside of the United States before, and although I consider myself worldly, I must admit that my view of medicine is not.

I've met practitioners from other countries who were skilled, even renowned, but I've never thought about the delivery of medical care through any lens other than my American one. And, I'm a little embarrassed to admit, I was skeptical of Dominican medical care at first.

We drove to the clinic, a modest building about a mile from our cabin. The care providers included a couple of nurses and a nurse practitioner; the doctor wasn't in that day. The clinic was small but relatively clean by American standards. I know that sounds kind of arrogant, but the clinic wasn't exactly like a typical urgent care center in the States. It was sparse by American standards, but the medical team was calm, confident, and professional. The clinic had air conditioning, which was nice; however, it had doors that didn't shut completely and at one point Jon saw a lizard sitting on a wheelchair. Luckily, I missed that, but by then I was so out of it that I might not have cared. There were a couple other people in the clinic but not many at all.

Jon's first impression was very *Americanized* as well.

"They looked surprised to see us, which made me very nervous about the kind of care we were going to receive," he recalled. "I was already apprehensive about any kind of medical treatment in Dominica. The first nurse we spoke to seemed a little uneasy about talking to us. We obviously weren't local residents and didn't have *the book* with us, so the process was not what they were used to. *The book* is something everyone in Dominica has. It's just a tablet like the ones we used to use in school to write essays. Each person has their own book with all their medical history recorded in it. Since Susan didn't have a book, the nurse had to start writing down all the info about her before they would examine her. It was a bit of a challenge, since it was all Susan could do to focus and the nurse spoke the usual Caribbean English, which is hard to understand at the best of times. I added information as needed to fill in the gaps."

I could barely keep my mind focused on the nurse's questions. She was so kind and patient. I'd start to answer a question and lose track of what I was saying, look to Jon, and he would finish my sentence. It was this weird joint conversation in which we were both speaking as if we were talking from the same brain because I couldn't articulate all the words myself. I remember that the room was a soothing yellow color and there was some light blue on the walls, too. I was dizzy and in pain. At one point, I even fought off tears. My mind was racing, but it wasn't the comfortable race of ideas that I was used to. It was as if I were struggling to keep my very essence present in the conversation.

If you've ever driven in a snowstorm or pounding rainstorm at night with your high-beam lights on, you know how it looked in my head: a constant attack of thoughts. When I talked to Jimmy about this later, he suggested that my fight-or-flight reflex had kicked into high gear. Knowing what I know now, I believe I was literally starting to fight for my life without even realizing it.

After the initial interview and once all the necessary information was collected, we were led into another room where I lay down and was given an IV by a grumpy-looking nurse. She seemed put out by us being there, which added to Jon's concern. Shortly after that, the nurse practitioner came to examine me. Her name was Eleanor and she was very thorough. Blood was drawn, urine was collected, the works.

Eleanor couldn't come to any conclusions or rule anything out without the results from the blood tests, but at that point we were all still thinking it was gastrointestinal. Our goal was to get me stabilized. We hadn't canceled our travel back to the States yet and I still believed that I might rally with some medical care. I don't remember this at the time, but Jon says that appendicitis was suspected but so was a stomach ailment. We couldn't be sure until a scan was done at the hospital in Roseau. At this point, no one was sure that a trip to the hospital was needed. Remember, the lone hospital was across the island, a one-hour drive away along a winding mountain road.

After a bit, I started to feel better. The IV was helping. My brain started to come back to life and the fog was clearing. I could focus, the images in my head slowed down, and I was a lot less confused. We were feeling more confident that maybe this really was just an intestinal issue. The nurses and nurse practitioner had warmed up to us and we were making casual conversation with all of them.

"At this point I felt like they did care about us," Jon said. "The grumpy nurse actually turned out to be very personable. We found out that she had a rental house just down the road and was curious how we found the place where we were staying. I told her about the website VRBO and suggested she put her place on the Internet. She made lots of notes about that. We also talked about her kids living in the United States and about the recent presidential election."

Jon asked one of the nurses what the process of payment was since we were from out of the country. She was surprised and said there was no charge for anything they did there. We were shocked and somewhat relieved. We were happy to pay whatever treatment cost and prepared to do so but had no idea how to navigate the Dominican health care system. We're also used to the nightmare of US health insurance practices. There was a simple humanity in the Dominican approach that was very refreshing.

The IV was working and I had to go to the bathroom. The nurse let me up and I kind of rolled over to one side into the fetal position and pushed my way up to a seated position using my elbows and the hand that didn't have the IV in it. I was still in a lot of pain, but the reverse pressure was helping and just having the fluids in me gave me energy that I hadn't had for the past few days.

Jon helped me navigate to the restroom with my IV pole and waited outside the door. Once I was done, I was washing my hands and the convulsions hit me full-on again. I felt like an electrical jolt had just struck my body. My arms and legs started jerking out of control and my teeth kept chomping on each other. I tried hard to stay upright by leaning against the door frame to steady myself.

The IV came out from the frantic shaking. It was like a slow-motion scene from a movie. The needle slid out of my skin. Blood spattered everywhere in the bathroom. And I mean everywhere. It was a mess. I called out to Jon in a staccato voice that didn't even sound like me and asked him to get the nurse. I was embarrassed that the bathroom was such a mess. I remember not wanting to be such a messy patient, especially after they had been so nice. Then I told myself that this was a medical clinic and that these professionals were used to all kinds of messes.

The nurse came, took one look around the room, and together with Jon, helped me get back to the bed. For a fleeting moment, I was really worried, but then my mind fogged up again and I lost all sense of time. I could hear talking going on around me, but it was slow and disjointed and didn't make sense. I knew I needed to pay attention and I had to fight to remain focused in real time. The blackness I'd seen earlier was back, but I refused to let my brain surrender to it. I could see it in the distance of my mind's eye, but I worked hard to turn my back to it and concentrate on what was happening around me. I concentrated with every fiber of my being to remain in the present.

I must have looked very confused and scared because the nurse held my hand. She looked right into my eyes and connected with my soul and said, "You're going to be all right." Despite the fog, her kind reassurances registered with me. Her eyes glowed with a warmth and confidence that was otherworldly, and I felt calmer. I was still confused, but I wasn't panicking. Someone was in charge. Someone would help Jon do what needed to be done. My brain was still very, very confused and fighting like crazy to remain in the moment, but the convulsions stopped and I was able to calm down.

From Jon:

"At this point I was getting very concerned. I knew this was something serious. I was concerned about my wife and that we weren't going to make our scheduled flight the following day. I was scared that we were going to be stuck with third-world medical care for quite a while. I had no idea what we would have to go through. I started to pace the room that Susan was in. The nurse noticed I was worried and tried to calm me down by reassuring me that everything would be okay. I wanted to believe her, but I could still feel myself going into preservation mode for me, but mostly for Susan."

The clinic medical team agreed that whatever was going on with me was beyond what they could treat. They called the local ambulance and then drew blood with the intent to transport it with me so that treatment at the hospital could get under way a little faster.

I knew Jon would notify the family of any changes to our travel plans, so I didn't worry about that at all. We agreed that we didn't want to worry the kids until we knew more about what was going on. The ambulance was called and on its way.

The "ambulance" turned out to be a van with a light on it. There was an oxygen tank inside, a bench, and a bed on wheels. The nurse told Jon to go back to our place at Citrus Creek to get a change of clothes for me. She said she would make sure the ambulance would be waiting for Jon along the road by Citrus Creek (which was on the way to the hospital) and he could follow it to the hospital in Roseau.

"I drove back to our cottage and had to calm myself down enough to think through what to pack," Jon remembered. "I made sure to get clean underwear and a couple other things I thought she may need. I also grabbed some food that I figured I would need during the wait. I drove back down the hill and the ambulance was waiting there for me. We began the hour-long trip to Roseau."

Meanwhile, the nurse and Jeffrey, the driver, helped me get into the ambulance bed. The nurse decided to go with me and carried an Igloo cooler with my blood samples in it. My head was facing the back door to the ambulance and I could see Jon's car through the window. I was worried that I'd throw up because I usually don't like riding backward, but I was in so much pain and starting to lose it again mentally that I figured throwing up was the least of my concerns. I think the nurse was afraid I was going to code en route. She tried to talk to me as if she was verifying my mental alertness. I finally said that I couldn't concentrate and asked if I could sleep. She agreed and told me to take a nice rest.

I drifted in and out of consciousness—I don't think I was sleeping. The blackness I'd seen before was creeping closer and closer every time I closed my eyes. It felt like it was becoming part of my consciousness, but I refused to let it take over even though it seemed to promise relief from my present circumstances. It would have been so easy to just drift off into that space because I didn't think I'd be in so much pain; but I was afraid to step into that void.

There was something inside me that would not surrender. It was taking a lot out of me, and my mental confusion and my physical pain were increasing. A lot. I needed an anchor to keep me in the present and in the light that I'd experienced in our cottage at Citrus Creek.

My anchor was Jon and he didn't even know it. In those rare moments, when I was aware, I looked out the back window to make sure that Jon was still following us. I was afraid of being separated from him because I knew he was scared for me. Not being able to stay close to the ambulance would have caused him even more anxiety and I didn't want to add to his burden. I was also very panicked at the idea that I'd lose consciousness and end up in the hospital with no one knowing who I was and no way for Jon to find me, literally and spiritually. I felt like I was on the brink of a choice that was being presented to me many, many times. I could remain in the present or move into the blackness and surrender myself to it. Simplifying my world and focusing on Jon in our little car enabled me to fight the blackness. Bottom line . . . I was trying to remain very calm for both of us.

As I mentioned before, the roads of Dominica are an adventure. It is a very mountainous island. Nothing is flat anywhere. The best roads on the island are barely wide enough for two cars to pass each other. They are constantly winding and either going uphill or downhill. The road from La Plaine to the center of the island, halfway to Roseau, is full of very large potholes, washed-out sections, rock slides, and construction areas. The potholes have potholes. In some places it is hard to dodge the potholes; there is nowhere to go but through them. I felt every single one of those twists, turns, and bumps. It was all I could do not to cry out.

From Jon:

"I stayed close to the back of the ambulance. We were both doing our best to avoid the potholes but still be expedient about our time. Some of the natives were in more of a hurry than we were. Apparently, there is no law or concern for giving emergency vehicles the right of way. No one pulled over for it and at least three other vehicles passed us on the way to the hospital. The ambulance had its emergency lights on, but I guess that doesn't matter. I was worried about my wife, worried the ambulance might be run off the road, and worried that my little car was not going to make it. Mostly I was concerned about what was waiting for us at the end of the ambulance ride."

From Adventure to Emergency

When we arrived at the hospital, the ambulance pulled up to the spot where ambulances unload the patients. Jeffrey and the nurse helped me out of the van and into a wheelchair. The double doors to the ER were different from what I expected. One side was plywood and the other was metal with a small window of glass. I took a deep breath and let Jeffrey push me in. Jon had to find a place to park in a small and crowded lot and then came into the hospital.

Princess Margaret Hospital was built in 1952. It's an eight-hundred-bed hospital and handles all types of medical care. An addition to the hospital was under construction at the time but was just barely getting under way.

The waiting room was very small and cramped. It was hot, dirty, and full of people who were hard to understand. The ceiling was full of holes and it looked like it was falling in. You could say that the whole building was in disrepair, especially by American standards. I was exhausted from the drive in and my mind was on high alert again. I could barely remember my name, but somehow, I felt compelled to be as alert as possible and an advocate for my own well-being. Jon stayed right by my side.

The original nurse from the clinic told me, through her calm smile and eyes, that everything was going to be fine. She said the same thing to Jon. Then, she disappeared with the cooler of my blood samples. We never saw her again.

We were told to go to the admitting desk. Jon wheeled me up to the desk while trying hard not to hit anyone else with the wheelchair. It was that cramped. I was asked the same questions and the same information was written down that the nurse at the clinic had already written and the admitting nurse was holding. Hmm . . . same questions, different medical staff, hurry up and wait, just like in the United States.

I couldn't stay focused on the conversation and Jon had to finish my sentences again. Then we were told to wait in the hallway to be examined. After about fifteen or twenty minutes we were talking to another nurse or doctor who asked the same questions and information that had already been written down twice. Her workstation was basically a closet with a desk and a computer. An examining table was next to it and jam-packed with a lot of other things. There was barely enough room to move around let alone get a wheelchair in there.

"Someone will come by to give you an IV," she said in a kind, soothing voice. "We've also scheduled an ultrasound to see what's going on." She smiled and left.

I was exhausted, in a lot of pain—virtually every movement hurt—and very foggy. I tried to pray. I tried my usual calming mantras. Nothing worked. I simply had very little left to give myself.

We were wheeled back into the hallway and then taken to another room that had a few beds in it. They were separated by curtains but were nearly touching each other. It was almost claustrophobic, and I felt bad for Jon. I had a bed to lie in, but he was trying to sit in a chair without disrupting the other patients in the room. The nurse's desk was positioned such that you had to basically crawl over it to get to the bed. In one of the beds was an elderly man who seemed to be gasping for air. He was surrounded by a lot of people we assumed were his family.

We updated the kids to let them know we were at the hospital but didn't have any details yet. Jon was taking the lead to text with them.

After we settled into the room, I had a few moments of clarity and emailed my boss to tell her I wouldn't be back at work until I could recover from whatever was going on. Our return to the States would be delayed by a few days. I tried to make light of my situation and sent a list of top priorities. She assured me that everything could be covered in the office and said to focus on getting well. She's a smart, faithful woman and said she'd be sending many prayers for healing my way and offered any help we needed. I expected that response and was glad to receive it. I also texted the chief financial officer/human resources leader at the company to find out about health insurance for emergencies out of the country.

Let's think about this another way . . . I, the person who had committed to staying in touch one hour a day while on vacation in a tropical paradise, was on the verge of experiencing the worst medical crisis of my life and I was concerned that I'd be dropping the ball at work. Talk about a misaligned mind-body-spirit! Looking back on it, I think the universe was working hard to get my attention. I just wasn't fully ready to surrender. Yet.

I never received the IV, but I was taken to have the ultrasound pretty quickly. I climbed onto a bed near the machine and was told by the nurse that the doctor was on the way. Then I was left alone. It felt kind of weird to be by myself. I still wasn't panicked, but I knew that something serious was going on. I dozed on and off. The blackness was still present and trying to grab my attention, but more in the distance.

After a time, two doctors came in. They spoke Spanish to each other, which I didn't understand. The female doctor conducted the ultrasound. She spoke English to me and apologized for the coldness of the gel and the wand. The male doctor watched the screen and waited at the foot of my bed. The woman doctor had read my file but asked me to explain a little more about how I was feeling. Once I started to talk, the male doctor smiled and said, "Ah, Americano. I'm so glad we're allowed to like each other now." It turns out they were Cuban. I agreed but must admit that they could have been mortal enemies of America and I would have welcomed any help they could give me. I was that miserable.

I've had ultrasounds before and while they can be uncomfortable, they've never been painful. I also have a high tolerance for pain. Like I said, I've given birth naturally twice. But, I have never, ever, ever experienced the kind of pain I felt during that ultrasound. To get the pictures she needed, the doctor had to press hard into my abdomen several times. I started to cry—I didn't cry out, but I absolutely gasped each time. Tears streamed down my face and I almost came off the bed. I stayed as still as possible and tried to focus my mind on anything that would take away the pain but to no avail. At one point, the doctor apologized a few times and looked like she wanted to have a good cry, too. Same with her colleague. Then, all at once, it was over. She put down the wand, talked to the male doctor, and then looked me straight in the eye with sympathy and concern.

"I'm diagnosing appendicitis," she said in her heavily accented English. "We'll contact the surgeon and get this taken out."

I was both relieved and scared. I was glad to have a diagnosis but worried about having surgery in Dominica. My medical care so far had been expertly given, highly professional, compassionate, and efficient. Surgery was another thing entirely. I'd literally be unconscious and at the mercy of people whose language I could barely understand in a hospital that wasn't anything like I was used to and without any support for Jon. After taking a few moments to process the news, I rallied, got dressed, and prepared to tell Jon that we'd be staying a little longer than expected.

Jon's time during my ultrasound was spent a little differently.

"I paced the hallway for what seemed like thirty to sixty

minutes," he said. "I asked a local man if he knew what time the gas stations were open till. He told me until at least 10:00 p.m. I knew I had to get gas to get back to the cottage across the island. I also walked outside to see if I could get a cell signal or wireless connection. While I was outside I could see across the Caribbean to a most spectacular sunset. I hadn't seen one like that for a very long time. I remember thinking that it was a sign that everything was going to be okay even though things seemed pretty dismal at the time.

"During all this time, I was holding on to hope that it was still an intestinal thing, but it was more hope than anything else. I really wanted to make the flight the following day so we wouldn't be stuck on the island any longer than we had to be, especially if Susan was sick. My intuition told me that it was something more serious, but I was still holding on to hope that it was an easy fix."

I told Jon that I had appendicitis and both of us just looked at each other. I was trying hard not to lose it because I didn't want Jon to worry any more than I knew he already was. I really had no idea what to expect next. I've never had an emergency of this caliber before. I was confident I could handle whatever came my way because I was raised to have that perspective, but I really had no idea what would happen to me.

Somewhere between being diagnosed by the Cuban doctors and telling Jon, some kind of survival instincts kicked in and I realized I needed to trust the universe to take care of me. The blackness faded further into the distance. I remained on high alert mentally; I couldn't shut that down at all. In fact, my mind had taken on a new sense of energy of its own and I had to really concentrate on trying to get it to slow down.

I was worried about Jon. I knew I'd have an entire medical team looking after me, but he was all alone. When we got married, we had a traditional service. When the Episcopal priest who married us got to the part that said "for better or worse, in sickness and in health," we pledged our devotion to each other. In that remote island ER, I realized that those weren't just words. They were real. Very real. It takes a strong partner to show up when it's easy. It takes a soul mate to show up when it's hard or when the outcome is unknown. Jon was right there. He showed up. He stayed, and he was my advocate and champion every step of the way. I knew I could count on him. I didn't have to surrender to that notion. I *knew* it. And I did count on him. My biggest worry? Who was Jon counting on? Who was going to be supporting him?

I was unable to pray for myself, but I was able to pray for Jon. I said a quick prayer that he'd find the support he needed to get us both through this.

"Once Susan told me that she had appendicitis, my heart sank," Jon recalled. "I knew we were now there for a while. She was going to have surgery in what seemed to me to be a third-world hospital. However, even though the facility seemed inadequate, the process was not taking very long—we were in the door and had a scan done in about ninety minutes."

Once we knew that it was appendicitis I emailed my boss to tell her I'd be out at least one week and told her that all updates would come from Jon. I wanted this off my plate. Again, *really?* Who cares about work at a time like this? Obviously, I did. Call it a sense of duty. Call it honoring a commitment. Call what it really was . . . a life out of balance.

I knew Jon would be updating the kids once we knew more. I couldn't handle much texting at that point because my brain was really, really foggy. Plus, I wasn't sure that I could say anything that wouldn't make them more worried than I knew they already were and I didn't want to add to their fears.

Once I was back in the room waiting to be admitted officially to the hospital, Jon went into planning mode.

"I knew I was going to have to make the drive back to the cottage that night no matter what time it was, and I needed to get gas in order to do that. I didn't have a place to stay in Roseau and I had to gather all our things anyway. On the way out of the hospital parking lot to get gas, I asked the gate attendant if I would be able to get back in when I returned later that night. He said, 'Maybe, maybe not.' I was thinking, 'Great, now I have some kid messing with me during a time I need it least.' He showed me the actual parking lot right next to the gate, and that was where I needed to park. I was back from getting gas quickly and Susan and I sat in the small room for a bit. The doctor came in and told us that Susan had appendicitis and that she would be admitted to the hospital and surgery would be done quickly. Shortly after that, she was wheeled to the hospital ward where she would be staying."

I was wheeled outside of the ER building into the Dawbiney Women's Ward, a twenty-six-bed building shaped in a cross, with most women in the long section. I was assigned to bed number three and if my two neighbors and I had reached out our hands, we could have touched each other. Each bed had a chair and a small nightstand/dresser next to it. The chairs were the old elementary school–style bucket seats with no padding. There were freestanding oxygen tanks set up between each bed. The room was true Caribbean style with louvred windows at the top of the walls and just below the ceilings, no screens, and only ceiling fans. There was no air conditioning. Privacy was maintained by pulling curtains that were anchored on steel pipes suspended from the ceiling. Usually curtains were left open to help with airflow.

There was a common bathroom that reminded me of those in my college dorm, except smaller. There were three toilet stalls. One was functional. One was semifunctional: the toilet seat was missing, but the toilet itself worked. One was out of order. Each stall had handrails to help users stabilize themselves. The stalls were made of wood and the doors were on springs that creaked and groaned each time they were opened or closed. The sound made me think of the bathrooms at a summer camp I used to go to. There was a large utility sink, some storage for stainless steel bedpans, a janitor's closet, three sinks, some large mirrors, and three shower stalls. There was no soap and no toilet paper. I learned later that it was customary for patients to bring their own.

There was also a small kitchen that looked like something you'd see in someone's home rather than the pristine institutional foodservice kitchen I'd expect in an American hospital. Also in the ward was a break room for the nurses, a nurses' station that was located right next to the entrance doors, and a mobile nurses' station that was wheeled into the middle of the ward and used for transition meetings between shifts. Visitors had a public restroom at their disposal.

The ladies in the ward each had carved out their own personal spaces by bringing in their own sheets. In fact, I was one of only a handful of women (the ward was full) who were using hospital-issued sheets and gowns. A television was blaring religious music and energetic sermons constantly. One woman was groaning almost nonstop as if she suffered from mental illness and seemed desperate for help. I was the only white woman in the ward at the time—patient or professional.

I was apprehensive about the conditions but realized quickly that my upbringing would serve me well. I've shared a room with someone for most of my life (sister, college roommates, spouse) and am blessed with the gift of being able to shut out ancillary background noise. Even with my mental state the way it was, I knew I could handle the chaos of being in the middle of a very busy hospital ward. I can sleep anywhere. I also am, generally speaking, pretty low maintenance when it comes to creature comforts. I like clean bathrooms, regular showers, and clean clothes, but otherwise, I'm generally not put out by conditions that are less than one or two stars. I'll eat just about anything. As a seasoned traveler, I don't freak out too much around lizards, spiders, and other bugs. I'm not a big fan of bats because I think they're a little creepy, and like I said before, I'm scared stiff of snakes, but I didn't figure that too many would be slithering in and out of the hospital.

Although I was anxious about the surgery, I realized that I really had no control over anything from that point onward. I was working hard to quiet my mind and to bear the incredible pain I was in. Once I was in the ward, I took stock of my surroundings and thought immediately about Jon. As much as I didn't want to be sick, I was glad it was me and not him. First, I don't want him to suffer. Ever. Second, I figured that I could withstand the conditions better than he could. He's a trooper, but his control needs are even higher than mine and he needs his space defined a little more than was available in the ward. Plus, he needs quiet to sleep.

From Jon:

"I looked at Susan and said, 'Are you going to be okay in here?' Of course, she said that she would be. My worries and concerns were growing by the minute."

One of the ward nurses soon came to collect more information. She started asking the same questions we had answered three times already. Jon became frustrated and snapped at her, but she stayed very composed and continued with her form. At the end of the form she looked at Jon and asked if he had any concerns about me staying there.

"By now I was pretty much at my wits' end," Jon recalled. "I told her I had many concerns, such as whether Susan would be able to rest here, if the surgeons would be qualified to operate on her, if she would be taken care of. Should I go on?"

The nurse gave him a small smile and calmly said, "No, that's okay."

I finally received the IV that had been promised to me in the ER. By that time, I was becoming dehydrated again. My eyes felt dried out and I was fading in and out and really wanted to sleep. I was having a hard time talking in complete sentences. Jon had to leave my area for me to get the IV. The nurse came in, introduced herself, and proceeded to find a spot to stick me with the needle. The only place she could find was at the top of my right hand. I was too dehydrated for anything in my arms to be usable. She put the port in place and started the IV drip. She opened the curtains and Jon was allowed back in.

Jon, who had already been texting with Jimmy and our daughter, Katie, a creative businesswoman, let them know what was going on. Obviously, they were concerned and distraught. They also jumped right in the deep end to support Jon.

Katie: You've officially freaked out Jimmy by not answering his text messages after telling him that Mom doesn't feel well.

Jon: I've been answering him. I'm on wireless now. Still waiting on surgeon. The room with everyone in beds is roasting!

Katie: Everyone's in beds in the same room?

Jon: Yes. Unreal.

Katie: Omg

Jimmy: I need to ask what's the word? How's Mom? I'm guessing she's having the surgery there.

Jon: Me too.

Jimmy: I'm worried but can only imagine how u feel. Keep your head up. As 3rd world as I'm sure it seems Mom is not the first person to get appendicitis there and won't be the last. This may just suck for a day or so.

I was still drifting in and out. At this point it was early evening. The hospitalist came in. His name was Dr. Robert and he was in charge. He was incredibly professional and did his best to assure Jon and me that everything would be okay. He had a voice that sounded like he was smiling all the time. Jon and I both felt better immediately. While everyone had been professional and competent, Dr. Robert exuded confidence. Although he didn't treat my appendicitis as if it were routine, he also didn't indicate that he suspected anything other than a typical procedure.

Dr. Robert examined me, brought in some kind of metal EKG device that was connected to my chest by suction cups to take a baseline reading, and said we needed to wait for the surgeon, who had been called and was on his way in. He said they expected to do the surgery that night and that the typical hospital recovery period for an appendectomy was twenty-four to forty-eight hours. Jon and I both were feeling better about things and felt that, with any luck, we wouldn't be here as long as we originally thought.

The surgeon arrived and, immediately, the nurses' demeanor changed. There was a definite air of purpose and action. Where they had been professional before, now they seemed on high alert, as if a higher level of seriousness had just been conveyed. The surgeon's name was Dr. Theodore. He came across as a very stern yet confident type and said that they would be operating shortly. His examination was thorough, and he clearly had read my chart. One of the things that struck me was his concern for my modesty. He seemed more concerned about it than I did, which hit me as kind of funny at the time. I mean, I'm the woman who said yes when asked during childbirth if a group of paramedic trainees could come in to witness the birth as part of their class! The fact that I was even thinking about this at that time tells you how far gone my mind was.

Dr. Theodore didn't stay long, but I heard him giving instructions to the nurses as he was leaving. I thought at the time that he seemed to be like other surgeons I'd known in the United States who had a God complex, but Jon and I agreed that we weren't put out. To our American mind-set, assertive medical care wasn't such a bad thing—especially given our uncertainties.

At that point, Jon started to relax a little.

A nurse came in and prepped me for surgery. She introduced herself to me and talked to me while she worked. She bathed me, shaved my body, and helped me change into a hospital gown. My feet were left bare. This all took some doing because I was in a lot of pain. Virtually every movement felt like I was getting punched or pinched in the abdomen. The nurse was so careful and so compassionate. That made me feel better.

The nurse told me that the Caribbean style of medicine relied on patients and family members to participate in the patient's care. I didn't quite get all that she said, but I did realize that there was a reason so many visitors were in the ward all the time. They were helping patients to bathe and changing sheets in addition to providing support. I remember agreeing with her that Jon and I would support that style of care but thinking to myself that I had no idea how to do that since it was just the two of us. I dismissed the conversation and tried to concentrate on the upcoming surgery.

Jon kept up separate text conversations with the kids, who were both at work, Katie in Chicago and Jimmy in Cincinnati. They started using our family nicknames as they kept up their e-chatter. Katie calls Jon *Pod*, which is short for *Padre*. We often call Katie *Litto* or *Mun*, which are short for *Little Munchkin*, and Jimmy's known as *Mur*, short for *Murray*. Just about everyone has a nickname of endearment in our family and we use them interchangeably with real names. When the kids were early teenagers, they asked us to use their nicknames only in private. Thankfully, they got past that phase quickly.

Katie: Ok. Do you want me to book reservations for you at a hotel closer to the hospital?

Jon: The guy where we are staying said he will help. I might be here all night anyway.

Katie: Ok. Let me know. I have all the information and no limit on my credit card :) I love you guys!!

Jon: What you could help with is our flight. I don't know if we need to cancel and reschedule. I can't call Delta from here. Would you be able to call them and find out our options?

Katie: Ok

Jon: I'll email you the info now.

Katie: Ok. It's canceled for tomorrow. The change fee was waived when I called back to reschedule with the hospital information. He couldn't just leave it pending without a new date to book on. You should receive a cancelation email. To reschedule we have to mention the same code and the record will come up.

Jon: Thank you!! That helps tremendously!! We'll know more in the next day or so.

Katie: Ok! Let me know what else you need help with

Jon: Thanks, Litto

Katie: Was she going back to work this week? Do you want me to email her boss?

Jon: We have been in touch with her boss. Covered there. I purchased trip insurance for this trip which I'm hoping will cover some of the additional costs. If I email it to you would you be able to look into it for us?

Katie: Yep.

Jon: I'm hoping it will cover some medical costs. This will be expensive. I'll get you the hospital info.

Katie: OK. Yeah, hopefully you will not have to pay up front. Keep all notes from doctors, medical records, receipts, any paper they give you. You will submit the claim when you get back. You are covered for extensions of the trip because this is a medical condition, under the trip interruption protection. You are covered up to $10k/person for the medical bill. Does that help?

Jon: You're the best, Litto!! You have helped so much tonight. All of those things ease my mind a lot. Can't thank you enough.

Katie: You're welcome, I wish I could be there with you guys but I'm glad I can still help. The family is thinking about you guys too. Give Mommy a big hug for me!

Jon: I was worried about how I was going to handle all those things. Now I don't have to. Ok I will.

Katie: I've got your back, Pod!

Jon: Yes, you do. Nice job. Thanks again.

Katie: Do you guys feel like you're in good hands?

Jon: Actually yes. Everyone has been very kind. Surgeons exude confidence.

Katie: Is Mom scared?

Jon: They are prepping her now and she is nervous.

Katie: (sad face) How long will it take?

Jon: Don't know.

Shortly after I'd been diagnosed, Katie was also able to get a hold of Hervé to let him know we would need some extra car rental time and possibly an extended stay at the cottage. Jon also called Hervé from a phone at the hospital. A nurse was very kind and let him use a phone in the office. He wanted to let Hervé know that we wouldn't be leaving at 5:30 in the morning the next day as originally planned. Once that was done, Jon kept up the texts with the kids.

Jon: Just spoke to surgeon. He expects to take it out tonight. No travel for a few days. Mom would like the family to know.

Jimmy: Ok. Good he's taking it out asap. Do you want me to tell the family?

Jon: You can check with Mun and decide who tells who.

Jimmy: Ok, Katie said she was helping u guys get a hotel near the hospital. U need any more help with anything or are u squared away?

Jon: I think we're good for right now. Thanks, Mur.

Once I was prepped, I rallied. I've had surgery before and Jon and I usually have a plan on what's going to happen afterward because it helps to reduce our anxiety. In this case, the potential complications were compounded by the fact that it was the middle of the night and I knew Jon had to drive back across the island in the dark to get to our cottage and pack up. I told Jon that if he needed to leave at that time, he should. I knew I'd be out of it for a while and that there was an entire medical team who'd be looking after me. It was one of the hardest things I ever did. I was scared, trying to make the best of it, and didn't want Jon out of range. Quite frankly, I also couldn't handle worrying about him driving around the island by himself in the dark. I was a mess.

He looked me square in the eye and said that he would absolutely not leave me. He also asked me if I'd leave if the situation was reversed, to which I replied, "Under no circumstances." We did agree, however, that once I was out of surgery, given the all clear, and back in the ward, he'd leave. I would be out of it for a long time after the surgery, and it didn't make sense for him to sit and watch me sleep when so much needed to be done.

The orderlies arrived, transferred me to a gurney, and wheeled me off to the operating theater, which was in yet another building. Jon followed behind. I remember looking up at the ceiling and then the sky and then the roof of the outdoor hallway and thinking that this wasn't really happening to me. At any minute I'd wake up and this would have been a dream. A vivid dream, but still a dream. No such luck. Jon and I said we loved each other, he kissed me, and I was wheeled into the operating theater. The surgery was supposed to take about forty-five minutes.

I almost cried right then and there once I was transferred from the gurney to the operating table. Pain was now shooting throughout my abdomen in what felt like one constant twisting motion that just kept getting tighter and tighter. It was as if someone was squeezing my insides—or giving me a charley horse, as we used to say when we were kids—and not letting go. I was scared, in pain, and trying so hard to be brave. I just wanted to break down, but I wasn't willing to concede to that.

My brain, which was so hyped up on my own hormones trying to keep me alive, kept telling me to stay vigilant and to be aware of what was happening so I could help myself. The blackness was creeping back in. It was as if a mist were trying to creep out of the void and draw me in. What I thought I could do about it at that moment is beyond me, but that's how it felt. Whether my usual control needs were still in place or I was literally a victim of my body's fierce fight to live, I can't say. What I know for sure is that I felt like I had to be very present in each moment and fight tooth and nail to remain so.

I was able to come around enough in my head to give myself a good talking to. My brain was both foggy and racing at the same time and I knew that I had to keep it together to help myself heal. I also knew that I had to surrender to the medical team and let them do their jobs. In that moment, thankfully, I realized that surrendering wasn't giving up as much as giving in to a higher power than me: Jon, the medical team, the universe. I simply was at the end of my ability to influence what happened next and had to trust life.

The operating theater was a windowless, air-conditioned room that was brightly lit. I was transferred to the operating table and a nurse named Bobbie took charge of me. I shivered, and she brought me some blankets. Then Dr. Robert came in, along with several people I didn't know. Dr. Theodore was still scrubbing. Dr. Robert said in a calm voice that they were going to remove my appendix and that they were all there to make it as easy on me as possible. He told me not to worry and came across as very reassuring. He wanted to be sure I knew who was in the room, and every person introduced themselves by first name as if they wanted to be my friend. I smiled and so did they. I also thanked them for taking such good care of me. They smiled again. It felt like they were angels whose only concern was my well-being and it felt good.

They started to strap me down to the table and the anesthesiologist sat down behind me. He said softly that his name was Johnson. I was starting to panic again and could feel my heart racing and my breaths become shorter. I was almost hyperventilating. The blackness that I'd been able to hold at bay was creeping closer and closer. Dr. Johnson told me to relax and then I said something that made him realize I had an American accent. He told me he was Cuban and said the same thing the other Cuban doctors did: "I'm so glad we're allowed to like each other now!" I remember telling him, "Dr. Johnson, we should have been allowed to like each other a long time ago." He laughed and placed the mask over my mouth.

My breath was still short and I wasn't going under as quickly as he wanted. I could see the mask on my face and knew what to expect, but my fear of the blackness that was filling my head was making me panic. I could see the blackness starting to encircle me and I was scared. It would have been so easy to just surrender to it and escape from my present circumstances. Something inside me, however, refused to do that and it showed up in my resistance to going under the anesthesia.

Bobbie came and held my hand and started stroking my arm to calm me down. She was a lifeline to me when I needed it the most. I felt like a child whose parent was waving a magic wand to make a boo-boo go away. I also felt like I had an angel present with me who was anchoring me to reality. It was almost peaceful. Dr. Johnson then started to take deep breaths in the same way he wanted me to. We were basically breathing together. I was still fighting the anesthesia because of my disrupted breathing, but I remember having a quick thought pop into my head again that I was protected by the medical team present. I needed to surrender to them as the rays of light I needed and let these people do their jobs. They would keep me safe. The next thing I remember, I was being transferred back into my bed in the ward.

The kids had gotten hold of our extended families to let them know what was going on. We're a tight-knit group and although they were worried about Jon and me, they rallied immediately to support the kids. One of my sisters, who was vacationing in the Dominican Republic at the time, offered to come to Dominica. She and her husband also looked into a medical evac back to the States and sent us the info. Another sister and my brother told the kids not to worry because I was "one tough cookie" and that if anyone in the family could handle something like this, I could. They stood ready to help in any way needed. Jon's mom reached out to him immediately and continued to take care of his cat, Mr. Fluff.

Despite all that help, Jon's experience while I was in surgery was intense. Not only did he have to hold it together for himself, by himself, but he had to keep texting the kids as well. He also texted his mother, whom Katie had nicknamed Mema, or Meem for short, when she was little, a name that's now used by all of us.

Jimmy: Any word on how long it'll take?

Jon: The nurse said about 45 minutes. It's been about 20 so far.

Jimmy: Wow. Maybe surgery there isn't as bad as I thought — that's pretty quick.

Jon: They have actually been very efficient here. Besides the sub-standard facilities and cleanliness they have been good.

Jimmy: That was and remains my biggest concern for all of this — contamination. Hoping nothing preventable happens because of it.

Jon: The surgery area looked sterile. Can't say that about the rest of the place.

Jimmy: The risk of surgery there is far less than the risk of flying home and having it done in the States in a day or two.

Jon: True. She was very sore. Still waiting.

Jimmy: Were u able to get all your guys stuff from the house?

Jon: I need to go back tonight.

Mema: Just talked with Katie. Not sure if u get this. Thinking of both of u.

Jon: Thanks, Meem. Not a nice experience.

Mema: Praying 4 surgeon to have steady hands. Keep in touch if u can. Love 2 u both.

Jon: Thanks, Meem. Surgery yet tonight. We'll be here until at least Thursday or Friday.

Mema: Thanks 4 up date. Mr. Fluff will be taken care of. Wish I could b with u. Not fun 2 b alone at this time.

Jon: Especially in these hospital conditions. Not the US for sure.

Mema: I know, that was my first thought. All I can say is I am praying God is watching over u 2

Jon: Thanks, Meem

Mema: Keep in touch

Jon: I will

Jon: She's in now. They said about 45 minutes. It's already been about 15.

Katie: Ok. Is it anesthesia?

Jon: Yes

Katie: What are you doing?

Jon: Sitting on a bench waiting.

Katie: Did you see any other cool animals besides birds and lizards?

Jon: Not really.

Katie: She's probably having some crazy dreams right now!

Jon: Could be. She was acting strange the last few days. This explains it. I keep losing Wi-Fi. I'll have to text you when she's out.

Katie: Ok, Pod. Love you.

Jon: Love you. Longest wait ever.

Katie: Still waiting?

I learned later that virtually everyone we know who knew of our situation was praying for us and sending positive energy. They also rallied their own prayer chains. I totally felt that love and support during surgery and afterward. I can't quite explain it, but once I got out of my own head long enough to let that peace envelop me, I felt so loved. It helped me keep the blackness at bay.

Jon's world during the surgery wasn't as peaceful as mine. In his words:

"I walked out to the car to grab my plastic bag that had a couple food items in it. I hadn't eaten since breakfast and it was now about 11:00 p.m. I brought the bag back with me and ate a few things on my bench outside the operating room. I was out there by myself.

Occasionally a maintenance person would walk by. If I walked closer to the ward area I could get wireless on my phone. I kept losing the wireless connection, so texting was a challenge, but at least I had a connection to family during the waiting.

"The first forty-five minutes came and went. An hour came and went. At that point I was getting scared and my mind began playing games with me. What if there were complications? What if something went wrong with the anesthesia? Susan doesn't handle drugs very well. What if she dies on the operating table? How would I tell the kids, being so far away? How would I get her body home? How would I live without her? I sat on my bench by myself and tried to stay calm.

"After about ninety minutes the two doctors came out. They both looked very tired and concerned. They looked for me and spotted me on the bench. I thought, 'This doesn't look good.' The surgeon did all the talking. He said that the surgery was done, and Susan was okay. The appendix had ruptured, he told me. He was very clear about how serious this was and could have been.

"I asked if she was stable and he said she was. I asked if she would be under the anesthesia for a while and he said she would be. I asked when I could come back in the morning and he said first thing. I thanked both of them and gathered my things. I texted the kids and my mom and told them the surgery was done. I provided a few details about the severity of it."

Jon: Surgery is done. Mom is stable but it was serious. Her appendix had already ruptured inside of her. There was a lot of puss and fecal matter inside her that they had to clean out. She now has a drainage tube in her to drain the infection and we will be here longer than expected. I'm heading back to the house now so will be out of touch for a while.

Jimmy: Wow

Jon: If she would have gone one more day, it could have killed her.

Jimmy: Yes, it absolutely could have. Glad she's ok. Did u talk to her?

Jon: No. She'll be under for a while. I'm leaving now.

Jimmy: Ok

Again, in Jon's words:

"I felt guilty leaving the hospital. The surgery was successful, but the situation was far from over. I knew she was going to have to spend the night in what looked like a MASH ward. I was very worried that she would be okay there alone. I was concerned she might have trouble coming out of the anesthesia. Would she be scared when she woke up? Would she be able to rest in that loud, hot, and seemingly unsanitary area? I had no choice. I didn't have a place to stay there and I needed to go back to get our things and make other arrangements anyway. I had to drive back and trust that she would be in good hands while I was gone.

"The drive back to Citrus Creek is not an easy one during the day let alone at 12:45 in the morning. The good thing was there weren't any other cars on the road. The bad part was there weren't any other cars on the road. If I had car trouble (a definite possibility with the car I was driving) or an accident, chances were good that I wouldn't have anyone to help me for hours. Plus, I was physically and emotionally exhausted. I started to drive and just focused on keeping my eyes on the road, remembering to stay left and watch for deep potholes. I started winding my way up the mountain.

"After about thirty minutes it started to rain. Now it's dark, raining, and I'm driving on an unfamiliar narrow, winding, pothole-riddled road and not even halfway back. I just kept my eyes on the road and kept going. I reached the roundabout, which was the halfway point of the trip. It is also the center of the island

and hub of all the roads there. That doesn't mean it is the center of civilization, however. There is nothing there. It also meant that the best part of the drive was over. The road from the roundabout to Citrus Creek was bad! This was where all the construction was. I kept my eyes on the road and kept going. I remembered certain points on the road, so I knew about where I was at various times.

"I made it back to the cottage about 1:45 a.m. I remember texting the kids to let them know I made it back. I also texted Susan and said, 'That was a close call. Love you.' I knew she wouldn't get the text until later and she may not even know that *close call* meant that she was lucky to be alive. I drank what was left of some red wine and one beer, thinking it might help calm me down. The events of the day had me pretty keyed up. I took a shower in the Banyan tree and then lay down to try and sleep. I just kept going over in my head what had happened. I also didn't know what else we were going to have to go through. I hardly slept at all and basically lay there and waited for the sun to come up."

Recovery in the Ward

I woke up briefly when I was transferred from the gurney back to my bed in the ward. I felt like my head was in a fishbowl of water. I heard conversation around me but couldn't really understand it. I also saw people hovering and checking my vital signs. And, I felt warm, reassuring hands move my body from one bed to the next, check my incision site, and make sure that the hand my IV was in was easily accessible. Otherwise, I slept.

Around 5:00 a.m., my nurse came in again to check my vitals. The staff seemed obsessed with my blood pressure, temperature, pulse, and blood sugar. I was awake and asked if I could get up to use the bathroom. I really didn't want to use a bedpan. I was incredibly sore and felt very weak and didn't know anything about my surgery or the seriousness of my situation. I don't remember if the nurse actually agreed to me getting out of bed, but I was already in motion, so she jumped in to help.

The act of getting out of bed took some doing, even with help from my nurse. First, I had to turn from my back to my right side, which was more like flopping my body over by sheer force of momentum. I had absolutely no abdominal strength whatsoever. The muscles of my midsection felt like jelly. Once on my side, I clutched the edge of the bed with my IV-free hand and then bent into a fetal position with my feet hanging slightly over the side of the bed. Then, I pushed myself to sit up using my right elbow on the bed because my hand was sore from the IV and it hurt to put pressure on it. I used my left hand to apply some reverse pressure to my lower right abdomen at the incision site. I could barely sit up. I remember thinking that I was glad I'd been trying to keep a fairly regular workout schedule, even though I'd fallen behind a little before this trip—hiking, weight training, spin, and yoga. I can't imagine having to do this with muscles that weren't used to moving!

The nurse was spotting me and helping me as much as she could in the cramped space. She'd moved the IV pole to the foot of my bed causing the plastic tubing to snake across my chest. I sat still for a few minutes. I was a little light-headed since I hadn't had any food in me for the better part of two days and had spent most of my time in bed. I didn't share this with the nurse, however, because I assumed it would pass and I didn't want to be forced to use a bedpan.

I grabbed the IV pole with my left hand to steady myself. I pushed on my abdomen with my right hand. The nurse grabbed me by the right arm and I managed to stand. The whole process took at least five long minutes. The concrete floor was cold and felt rough on my feet. After making sure I was steady the nurse leaned down and put on my sandals. She also grabbed a pair of undies for me as I was still naked under my hospital-issued gown from the surgery. We then started walking toward the toilets.

I didn't set any great land speed records. My steps were actually very small. I wasn't shuffling—the treads on my sandals and the roughness of the floor prevented that—but I could only handle walking about the length of one of my feet before I had to take a step with my other foot. Now, the bathroom was only about twenty-five feet from my bed. At the time, it might as well have been twenty-five thousand feet. Every single muscle in my abdomen was screaming out in pain from being stretched every which way to support both me in a vertical position and me walking. My pain meds dulled some of the pain, but they didn't get rid of it. I didn't ask for anything stronger because I didn't want to risk being incoherent. I refused to surrender, however. I gasped a few times but didn't cry out. Plus, there was no way I was going to be stuck in bed using a bedpan.

The bathroom area was open, with no doors until you got to the toilets and the showers, so it would be easy to enter. When we reached the bathroom area, the nurse pointed out a cart with about ten bedpans on it. She grabbed one and pointed me to the one stall with a toilet seat. She put the bedpan on the toilet seat and told me I had to pee into the bedpan so that they could keep track of my urine output. I was tired, hot, in pain, and a little un-steady on my feet. I thought I hadn't heard her right. This seemed a little archaic to me, but I was willing to go through these steps with the bedpan in order to use a toilet (at least I didn't have to pee in bed!). I didn't say anything, and she repeated herself and added "This is very important" for emphasis. I nodded my head to let her know I'd heard her. She asked if I wanted her to come in. I declined and said I wanted to try it on my own. She looked a little skeptical but agreed as long as I didn't lock the door.

The bathroom stall was about one and a half times the size of the usual stall of an American women's public restroom. Let's think about that a minute. There I am, less than ten hours postsurgery, with tubes hanging out of me, an IV pole on wheels trailing me, and a midsection that doesn't seem like it could support me try-ing to relieve myself while balancing on a metal bedpan perched on top of a toilet seat, all in what quickly became a very cramped space. It was surreal. I mean, you just can't make this kind of stuff up.

When I was finished, I realized that there wasn't any toilet paper in the stall. In fact, there wasn't a toilet paper holder in the stall. Just a small shelf. I asked the nurse for some toilet paper. She'd been looking in on me and for a brief second, her face showed some surprise rather than its usual serene glow. She brought me some and I was able to finish my business and step out into the room. I was exhausted. The nurse brought me some soap. I washed my hands and then she helped me into my undies. Before taking me back to my bed, she checked my bedpan, noted something on a chart, and then put it in an industrial-size sink to be sanitized before going back into the rotation for use again. Next time, I'd have to grab the bedpan myself and, when finished, let the nurse know so she could check everything and update her charts.

I eased my way back into bed by reversing everything I'd done to get out of bed. I'm not sure which was more painful, but I did it and said a quick prayer of thanksgiving that since I'd made it through the bathroom routine once, I would be able to avoid being locked down in my bed. I was proud of myself. Yay!

I knew Jon was going to be worried about me, so I sent him a quick text to let him know I was okay. Then, in a moment of lucidity, I thought of seven things that I'd forgotten to tell my boss about the day before and I shot her a quick email, said I was checking out, and told her Jon would be doing all communicating from then on. It was 6:00 a.m. Dominican time, 5:00 a.m. Eastern time. She answered when she got into the office that all was well and kindly said, "Let's talk about what's really important … How are you? How is your recovery going?" She also said she'd follow up with Jon and repeated her offers of help. Her biggest concern remained my well-being. She was so kind!

I knew that the incredibly talented team at my office would be doing a fantastic job. Mostly, I was concerned that I was working on something that they might not have had line of sight to. We were beyond busy, and I didn't want them to get caught short because I had failed to bring them into the loop on something. My boss was amazing. She seems to thrive in an atmosphere that requires quick problem solving. As I've mentioned, she is a woman of great faith and I knew that she wanted only the best for me and for Jon.

Still . . . the fact that less than ten hours out of surgery I was thinking about work reveals just how messed up my priorities were at that time. I absolutely do not judge anyone who is a dedicated employee. On the one hand, I think work kept popping into my head because during all the uncertainty and madness I was experiencing, it was logical. I knew what needed to be done and could actually do it. There was comfort in thinking about work during a time in which my brain was mostly full of psychedelic imagery swirling around trying to steer clear of the blackness void.

I'd like to believe that thinking about work was needed at the time. On the other hand, the fact that work stuff kept bubbling up to the front of my very confused mind should have been a red flag. Somewhere, my brain must have gotten the message because I suddenly stopped thinking about work. It was as if a switch went off in my head and work just vanished. That was an important step in my recovery. It was time to focus only on me.

The nursing shifts were about to change and there was a lot of activity in the ward. Virtually every woman in the ward was visited by her *girl posse* to change linens and help with bathing, grooming, and changing clothes. That means that there were two to four women visiting nearly each of the twenty-six women in the ward at that time. That's a lot of activity! It was chaotic, but also had its own weird sense of peaceful flow about it. There was a positive, healing energy that came from every one of the people present. I was alone in my bed, but I didn't feel lonely. I was tired, a little confused about what had just happened to me, and in a lot of pain. You'd think I'd be scared. On the contrary, I felt like I was surrounded by this powerful life force filled with love and compassion. In fact, several of the visitors smiled and nodded at me as they walked by my bed.

During this time, the nurses were updating charts and meeting with the next shift. Dr. Theodore came to check on me. It was the first time I remembered talking with him since his presurgery exam the day before. He called my nurse over and pulled the curtains. He asked me if I knew what had happened. I told him that I'd had my appendix out but didn't know anything else. I asked him how everything went.

The simple concern he showed on his face in that moment is something I'll always remember. He looked me straight in the eyes and started to tell me the truth about what had happened. He was very concerned with how I'd take the news. Before he gave me the details, he had the nurse move to stand on the other side of my bed so that they were flanking me. It was as if they were embracing me without touching me.

Dr. Theodore told me that my appendix had ruptured and that infection had filled my abdomen. Essentially, the contents of my appendix and my colon had spilled into and contaminated my body cavity. He also said that the point where my appendix joined my large intestine was necrotic (which means it had already died—he was ever the doctor!) and gangrene had already set in to that area. I had peritonitis and was septic. He also said that I was within hours of dying if I'd delayed getting to the hospital any longer.

As he was going over the details, he watched me closely to see if I understood what he was saying and to see if I was going to panic. He spoke Caribbean English and was sometimes hard for me to understand and I asked him to repeat a few things from my story. However, as exhausted as I was from my first trip to the bathroom and as fogged as my brain still was from the drugs and the events of the past two days, my mind cleared for a moment and I was able to follow exactly what he was telling me. Word. For. Word.

The seriousness of my situation hit me like a ton of bricks. I'd almost died. I'd. Almost. Died. What had been my world might have been continuing without me. At that very moment, instead of Jon packing up our stuff and relocating to the other side of the island to be near me, he could have been planning for my body to be shipped back to the States. He could have had the impossible task of telling the kids and our families what had happened. I had an entire medical team watching over me. He was alone. What he'd gone through on my behalf was almost overwhelming to me and I was filled with such a powerful sense of love for him.

As I listened and then watched the doctor check my incision site and the site of the drain he'd left in, I was overcome with such a sense of gratitude to the universe for putting my life in the capable hands of this medical team. I was thankful for the doctors' expertise and that of everyone in the hospital who was watching out for me. I was thankful for the many people who were praying for me. I was humbled and felt choked up with emotion.

"Thank you," I whispered to Dr. Theodore as I put my hand on his arm. He seemed a little startled, but smiled and nodded.

Dr. Theodore told me that because of the seriousness of my situation, I'd likely be in the hospital until the end of the week—another three to five days—and that while he'd be checking in on me at least once a day, Dr. Robert would also be checking on me. I asked him what I could do to help myself and he said I should walk as much as possible. I knew from previous surgeries in the United States that walking was an important part of healing. I'm not very good at staying still, so I was very relieved to hear Dr. Theodore's suggestion and quite frankly, glad to have something to do. It might take me at least five minutes of pain each way to get in and out of bed, but I was bound and determined to walk.

Once again, texts were the family lifeline as Jon brought everyone up to speed. At this point, he was still on the other side of the island. We had exchanged some texts but had not yet talked with each other.

Jon (to both kids): I heard from mom this morning. She said she made it through the night ok. Probably better than I did. I need to take care of some things here and then I'll make the hour trek back to the hospital. She has her phone, so you may hear from her. I'll let you know more as I get info.

Jimmy: Ok, thanks. I slept terribly too. Very worried about her and you. Did they have to cut mom open or do they have microscopic abilities.

Jon: Not sure. I think because the appendix ruptured they had to make a larger incision. The doctor just told mom the base of her appendix was dead.

Jimmy: Wow. Everything else ok? Her large intestine have any disease too?

Jon: They didn't say anything about that.

Katie: Ok. Let me know if there's anything you need.

Jon: K Litto.

From Jon:

"I may have gotten an hour or two of sleep before I got out of bed. I looked at my phone and saw a text from Susan about 5:00 a.m. She said she was doing okay and had been up and walking already. That was a huge relief to me since I was feeling guilty about leaving her at the hospital. I was glad she had come out of the anesthesia and was doing okay. I responded back to her but don't remember what I said. I think I mentioned something to her about the severity of the appendix when they went in to remove it. She hadn't heard from the doctor yet as to what had happened. Shortly after that I believe the doctor came in to talk to her and explained what happened. I still don't think she comprehended how serious her condition was and that she could have died from it. That would come later.

"At some point during the morning she texted me and told me that there was no hurry for me to get to the hospital, since all she was doing was lying there in the bed. Even in a time of pain and discomfort she was still thinking about me. She has always put me and the kids first and even at that time she was doing the same thing."

Jon: That was a close call. Love you!

Me: Made it through the night. Can you bring me some bottled water when you come! Love you!

Jon: Good!! I've been worried about you there. You were a very sick girl. Did they tell you it had already ruptured? Yes on the water.

Me: I'm fine. OMG! That's serious but it does explain why they're keeping me pumped with antibiotics. No communication from doctor yet. Nothing to eat or drink yet but I want to.

Jon: Be ready. Take your time.

Me: No rush to get here at all. I'm sleeping a lot. Looks like you'll be touring Roseau.

Jon: Yes it does. They said you also have a drainage tube in you to let the infection drain out. They said another day and it would have been life-threatening. Trying to go home wouldn't have worked too well. The down side is they said it means longer stay.

Me: Doc just came and said the base of the appendix was dead, which is very serious. No food or drink today for me.

Jon: You must have been in pain for a while. Didn't you feel anything before this?

Me: I did, but it wasn't anything that couldn't be attributed to muscle aches. Well . . . I always say go big or go home. Of course, being home would be better right now.

Jon: Yes it sure would be. Do you want any clothes, toiletries, etc.?

Me: Yes. I have a red bag. Can you buy some extra toothpaste and soap, put in the bag toothbrush, toothpaste, comb, clean undies x 2, hardback book, shampoo and TP. Also nightgown, charger plus Mophie charger which is in a small zipper bag in my backpack. No shorts. I still have a drain in me and nothing can go over it. Also Ziploc for soap.

While I fell asleep at the hospital, Jon was on the other side of the island at Citrus Creek getting things organized at the cottage. Life wasn't so smooth for Jon.

"I ate breakfast and began to clean up the kitchen. There was some food that had to be tossed. Our original meal plans had been disrupted by the medical emergency. During breakfast I checked a couple things on my iPad. I always checked email, the weather at home, and the temperature inside our house at home. Before we left on the trip I bought a little thermometer that connects to the Internet so I could see what the house temperature was while out of the country. I always try to plan for the unexpected when we're gone and since it was winter, I didn't want to risk a problem with the furnace that might lead to frozen pipes. I thought that if the furnace had trouble I would be able to see by the house temp. I checked that app on my iPad and of course the house temperature was down to fifty-two degrees. Just what I needed today!

"I texted my mom and she was able to stop by the house on her way to work. She verified that the circulating pump was running but there was no flame. Most likely the thermal coupler. I texted our neighbor, who was able to go over and replace the thermal coupler for me and get the heat back on. I always keep a spare by the furnace. Saved by a good friend/angel once again. Good thing I thought of the thermometer or else the house would have frozen up."

In another moment of grace, two dogs who lived at Citrus Creek came up to see Jon.

"Citrus Creek had a couple pups we had seen while we were there. They were always hanging around the main restaurant area. They were friendly pups, but they never seemed to leave the main area. They were usually lying on the pavement outside. I had played with them a few times when we passed by the main restaurant but had never seen them by our cottage. When I had gone out to fix myself some breakfast they came up to see me. The male lay on the porch of the cottage while the female stayed close to me. She just looked up at me and wagged her tail the entire time. It was as if she knew I needed to have her near me to help calm me down. She was right, although they may have also been there to get into the smelly garbage that was in the can. In either case, it was comforting to have them there with me. I still like to think they were there because they sensed I needed them."

After breakfast Jon went down to meet with Hervé. He explained what had happened. Hervé was as shocked as we were as to the severity of the situation. Jon and Hervé talked a bit about what had happened and then Hervé helped Jon find a place to stay in Roseau. Hervé made a couple of recommendations and called the places to help set up the reservations. He was also able to extend the rental of the vehicle for as long as we needed it.

"I told him how much we enjoyed our stay there and how much I appreciated all his help with our medical emergency," Jon said. "He was gracious accepting the accolades, but also acted like it was just part of how he treated all of his guests.

"When we booked a place to stay after we decided to go to Dominica, one of the reasons we chose Citrus Creek Plantation was so if we needed help with anything in a wild and foreign country we would have someone to talk to. It sure came in handy!"

Once the life details were taken care of, Jon went back up to the cottage to get things packed. He organized all our belongings and was getting bombarded by texts. Between texts with the family who were obviously concerned about me, our neighbor checking in on the furnace, email from my office . . . it took Jon a couple of hours to get things packed. Jon tossed everything into the car and started to make the hour-long, pothole-laden, mountainous trip back to Roseau. At least it was daylight this time.

Katie: Love you, dad.

Jon: Love you, Litto. Hervé helped me get a room closer to the hospital and we can keep the rental car longer. I think we're on track.

Katie: He's so nice

Jon: He is. They all are.

Katie: Are you back at the hospital yet? I'm trying not to bug you

Jon: Just got everything packed and am leaving now.

Katie: Any updates worth sharing?

Jon: We're good here Litto. Tell the troops they can calm down now.

Katie: Roger that. Keep me posted.

Roseau is a typical Caribbean island town. Once you get into the main town area, the roads are very narrow and there are a lot of people on the streets, a lot of traffic, and groups of people from cruise ships walking around. It is extremely hard to navigate in a timely manner and without side swiping another vehicle or a person. Cars will just randomly stop in the street, which means you have to wait until oncoming traffic stops (which it never does) or you take your chance to try to get around. There is barely enough room for a single car at times, let alone two cars passing each other. The bus drivers have no fear and will run you off the road. It's not a pleasant place to try to get around by car. Fortunately, Hervé told Jon about a couple of easy ways to get past some of the craziness. They came in handy for getting to the hotel.

Jon's first stop was the hotel that Hervé helped book. It was called the Castle Comfort Lodge and was both a boutique hotel and a diving center. Jon learned that Hervé had explained my situation to them and noted that we weren't sure how long we'd be staying. The owner of the hotel made sure we had a ground-level room so I wouldn't have to walk up steps once I was released. At that time we thought Saturday might be our last day in town and the owner confirmed that staying until Saturday wouldn't be a problem.

Jon was greeted warmly at the hotel. After receiving such genuine care from Hervé, Jon was starting to feel like he wasn't so alone. The hotel owners and guests took that up to a whole new level.

"When I made my way through Roseau and found the little hotel, they were waiting for me," said Jon. "The people at the front desk were very friendly and immediately asked me how my wife was. They checked me in to my room. I dumped all my things in the room, then got connected to wireless so I could text Susan. I told her that I had checked in and that I would be there shortly, but I might have to get something to eat first. She told me to take my time. I went to the bar that was just outside my room and had lunch. I was very tired from no sleep the night before and making the stressful drive back to Roseau. I was also still very worried about Susan."

Meanwhile, the kids were doing all they could to stay on top of things and support their dad, including adding in some humor when possible.

Jon: Just got a room. Packing a bag for her and going there soon.

Katie: Don't forget face wipes and deodorant! She can get stinky. Clean undies? I'm glad you feel better. Jimmy and I are still worried, but it makes me feel better to know you're better. I'm glad I was helpful last night. I'm good in crisis situations and panic afterwards.

Jon: Got the undies. How is the rest of the family gab?

Katie: They're sending good thoughts and positivity. Stay the course, keep the faith and all that.

Jon found his way back to the hospital using the route Hervé suggested, which bypassed a lot of the back alley–type driving in Roseau.

"When I went back into the ward, Susan was there and looked pretty good considering all she had gone through," Jon said. "The ward was still hot, but the afternoon crowd hadn't arrived, so it wasn't too noisy yet. We talked a little about what had happened with the ruptured appendix. It still hadn't sunk in for her that she could have easily died had we not gone to the clinic when we did. I told her about gathering all the things, my little hotel, and so on. After a while we kind of sat there and soaked it all in. She was tied to the IV and was receiving painkillers and heavy doses of antibiotics."

The next couple of hours we tried to digest everything that had happened to us. We were still pretty much in shock about it all. I took periodic walks, which Jon did with me. I also dozed on and off due to the painkillers and general lack of sleep. Every time I woke up, Jon was sitting by my bed. He never left. He got in trouble once for using the nurse's bathroom instead of the public one, but he still never left my side. I was very woozy and not altogether coherent. While I dozed, Jon texted the kids.

Jon: Sitting with mom now. She's doing much better. She looks a lot better. Not much anyone can do at this point. She just needs to rest up.

Jimmy: Really glad to hear that. Thanks for the update. I've been a mess today. How are u? Can I help u with anything?

Jon: I'm good. All settled in. Over the initial shock of it all. Why have you been a mess?

Jimmy: Just anxious as hell. I know how serious this is and am working myself up. Glad she's recovering well, though, that's good news.

Jon: The surgeons seemed very good. I was relieved when I met them.

Jimmy: That's good.

Jon: I think we're on track. The next day or so should tell us for sure. Just wish we were home.

Jimmy: I wish you were too. She's pretty resilient. Will keep hoping for the best.

Jimmy: Once someone is septic things are already VERY bad. What mom had was called peritonitis. It is an infection of the inside lining of her gut, caused by some pretty bad bugs in her bowels. Her chills and convulsions were very typical for that kind of infection. Sepsis is tough to treat, so if not recognized right away and acted upon it can be a few days before they might pass away. There are all kinds of sepsis and sterilization protocols in the US that we follow, and I was afraid that down there they didn't have medicine at the caliber they do here. But it sounds like they do and she is responding appropriately to all the treatments and care.

Katie: Dad, do you want me to come down there?

Jon: Sure Litto, we can go hiking. Sitting with mom now. She's doing much better. She looks a lot better. Not much anyone can do at this point. She just needs to rest up.

Katie: That's good!!

Jon: Not sure if you're serious about coming here. Actually you're way more useful at your command post.

Katie: I am serious, but I will do whatever you want me to do to be most helpful. I still have a key to your house too if you need me to ship anything.

Jon: I think we're all settled in. I feel much better about things now. You were a huge help last night. Now we just wait for mom to heal enough to travel.

When Jon got back to the hotel he made his way to the bar, had a couple of beers, and ate dinner. The bar area was next to the water with a very nice view.

"I felt guilty coming back to a nice hotel with air conditioning, a waterfront view, and a bar while Susan was stuck in the hot, noisy, and crowded hospital ward and stuck full of needles. The bartender was a local guy from Dominica. After a while he and I hit it off. He was a very nice guy with a big smile. He was an easy guy to like right off the bat. I explained to him why I was there and he was very sympathetic and caring.

"After a while a young guy sat next to me. We started up a conversation. He was a twenty-six-year-old guy from Seattle named Trevor who came to Dominica to do some hiking, diving, and general adventure seeking. As it turned out, he had been in the financial industry since he graduated from college. He decided to leave it and join the Peace Corps. This was his adventure before going. He also was very sympathetic and genuinely concerned about Susan. After a while I went back to my room. It was only about 9:00 p.m. but I was exhausted and crashed hard for the night."

I was worried about Jon. A lot. I was so relieved that he had his own angel team watching out for him at the hotel. The kids, of course, were watching out for him, too. We have an amazing extended family and they were all doing everything they could to support both of us. Jon, however, was all alone. At the end of the day, he had to eat alone and face an empty hotel room not knowing what was going on with me. As he was describing the people he met along the way, I got a warm feeling inside. I knew that no matter what happened, he wouldn't have to be by himself.

Stepping into the Light

There's one part of this story that I haven't shared in detail yet. Even though I lost sight of it for a bit during the initial crisis and a few times afterward, this one thing became the foundation for my recovery: I knew I wasn't going to die before I ever set foot into my first medical stop at the clinic.

Pause. Reread that sentence.

I knew I wasn't going to die before I ever set foot into my first medical stop at the clinic.

The emotions, the chaos, the blackness, and the fear were real, but I knew I wasn't going to die. I had no idea what that meant, but I knew it wasn't my turn to die. This wasn't a sixth sense or a premonition. It was real—the kind of pure truth that most of us long to feel but are afraid to believe.

After my first set of convulsions when Jon and I were still in our cottage, we were trying to decide whether to go to the local clinic. You already know this. I've described feeling like I was watching our conversation from a distance. I've described the inky blackness that was creeping closer and closer. That was true. What else happened is something I didn't share with Jon at the time. It was also true.

As we were talking, it was as if I had two brains, each working at the same time. One was in conversation with Jon and feeling every bit of the fear, confusion, pain, and uncertainty I've described.

The other part experienced a clarity of purpose like I've never felt before. My fog not only ebbed, it was nonexistent. There was no blackness. There was no pull to surrender to an easier path. I was floating above the room looking down on Jon and me, not sitting on the bed. The closest I can come to describing it is this: If you think back to a dream sequence in a television show or movie where the main characters are given a chance to watch their lives taking place from inside the dream, that's what it felt like.

I wasn't scared. In fact, I felt strangely comforted. For a fleeting moment, I wondered what was going on, but then I found myself cradled in light. I wasn't pulled toward or away from the light. I was surrounded by a bubble of light. My brain was perfectly clear. I wasn't in any pain. I could hear, see, smell, and feel. I had fresh breath, not the yuck of sickness. All of my senses were engaged.

The light was beautiful and warm. It felt the way the sun feels on a perfect day—a warmth that starts at the top of your head and spreads all the way to the tips of your toes. I wasn't standing up, though. I was cradled in what felt like loving arms. It was gentle and firm at the same time and I had no fear of falling. I could feel an expression of serenity on my own face and in my mind. It felt like the kind of security I've always imagined a child is feeling when they're sound asleep in their parent's arms.

It was peaceful and joy-filled and energizing all at the same time. I had no sense of time. I could have been in that moment for ten seconds or ten days. I had no idea.

I smelled all the outdoor smells I love at the same time. The freshness of spring right after it rains. The crispness of fall when the leaves start to change. The clean scent of a sunny winter day after a fresh snowfall. The salty fragrance of the beach at high tide.

I heard the song of birds and the pulse of the surf. I could see rays of light peeking into my peripheral vision. I felt the breeze on my face. I was warm, but not hot. There were no shivers or convulsions. Just peace. And strength. And comfort.

I felt rested. I felt whole. I felt the purest form of unconditional love that I've ever experienced. It was at the same time one moment and every moment. I could feel myself smile. I was supposed to be in this moment right now. I wasn't being rewarded for anything. I was worthy just the way I am. I mattered. I was enough simply by *being*.

Then, in the lightness of being, I heard a voice that wasn't male or female. It started out as more of a thought inside my head that my brain "heard" as a voice.

"You are not going to die," it said gently. "It's not your time. Trust me. You are enough and you're going to be okay."

The voice went silent, but the message was clear. It was not my time to die. Not a question popped into my head. I accepted the words as fact, but I had no idea what was going to happen next.

Suddenly, my two experiences converged, and I felt myself rejoin the conversation Jon and I were having about the clinic. All the pain and anxiety of my physical state returned in full force, but I still felt so loved and protected. I didn't tell Jon what had just happened to me—this battle between darkness and light, with my light winning. I didn't disbelieve it, I just couldn't explain it easily. Also, I was worried that he might be freaked out a little by it and I needed him to keep it together for both of us.

Many a book and sermon have been written about out-of-body experiences. In every case I've ever read, the experience wasn't dependent on a person's beliefs, level of faith, or connectedness to the universe. The experience, like mine, simply happened during a time of extreme uncertainty and choice and brought a sense of peace.

For me, that peace was an underlying sense of calm in my soul. My mind was racing, my body was wreaking havoc on itself, and my spirit was being tested in many ways. I couldn't even pray for myself—something that has never happened to me as long as I can remember. But, I knew with certainty that I'd get through whatever was coming my way. The blackness was not going to win. It was as if all my experiences and all the traits I'd acquired along the way had been conspiring my whole life to see me through this moment.

With all this in mind and as I look back, my remaining days at Princess Margaret Hospital took on a new significance. I wasn't out of the woods yet and I had still some important work to do of my own. But I had a touchstone to come back to when things really got tough.

Being a Patient
Requires Patience

By Wednesday morning, a day and a half postsurgery, I was familiar with the routine of the ward. In the wee hours of the morning, the girl tribes came in to help friends and family. Then, the doctors and nurses made their rounds. Right before work, which seemed to start anywhere from eight to ten o'clock in the morning, adults came by for social hour to visit patients. Around lunch, friends and family working in Roseau dropped in to eat with their loved ones. Midafternoon, children and grandchildren stopped by to visit after school. Dinner was usually pretty quiet, but then from seven to ten o'clock at night, the final wave of visitors arrived. At least three times per day, a cleaning crew came in and disinfected the floors and cleaned the bathrooms. They also disinfected beds as patients were released so they'd be ready for new ones. Amid this, we all continued to receive medical care.

The nurses were checking my vital signs every hour on the hour. They seemed obsessed with my temperature, blood pressure, and pulse. They backed off on the blood sugar checks, which meant fewer blood draws, but I was running a low-grade fever of ninety-nine to one hundred degrees and they were trying to figure out why. Also, I had broken out in a hive-like rash, but this I attributed to the soap used to wash my hospital-issued sheets. I have sensitive skin and this kind of reaction isn't uncommon for me. Dr. Robert, who was checking in on me regularly, noticed the rash and asked me about it. Since it was gone the next time he checked on me, we didn't think much more about it at the time.

I was receiving four syringes of medicine every few hours. Three were filled with antibiotics and were huge—one looked to me to be the circumference of a quarter. The medicine was administered through the port in my IV. A painkiller was given directly into my backside. I'm not squeamish around needles (thank goodness), but I also don't take medicine much stronger than aspirin, so I felt kind of like a human pharmacy.

Even with all that pain medicine, it was still a struggle for me to get in and out of bed, but I was forcing myself to walk around for five minutes every hour or so. I still couldn't walk very fast, but I was walking on my own with my IV pole and could ease myself in and out of bed without a nurse.

The ladies in the ward were all watching out for me as I walked up and down between the rows of beds. One woman, whose bed flanked the door to the bathroom, stopped me at one point as I made my rounds because I had slipped my feet into my sandals and didn't bother to strap them. She told me I should get some flip-flops to make it easier to walk around. She was genuinely concerned for my safety.

As I walked, I tried to respect everyone's privacy. This is kind of hard in an open ward. Occasionally, I'd catch the eye of another patient. We'd smile. She would usually nod or raise her eyebrows in that questioning way to see how I was doing. Sometimes our different forms of English created a barrier. We were able to communicate anyway in that secret language that women have with each other that says, "I'm your sister and I care."

The head nurse on day shift was a force to be reckoned with. She was smart, kind, and demanding all in one. Every day she clearly had a mission to keep the ward running as smoothly as possible and she wasn't afraid to bring down the hammer (gently) if needed to maintain the highest standards of patient care. I watched her as she moved from bed to bed, managed people, and ran the ward. She always exhibited the highest degree of professionalism, but it was truly all about patient care.

She was never assigned to be my direct caregiver, but a few times, she filled in if needed or watched over a newer nurse as she was checking my vitals. Nevertheless, she wasn't afraid to scold me when she felt the need. Although my routine had been to walk every hour, by Wednesday I was starting to get a little stiff and sore lying in bed all day, so I tried to walk more frequently. The doctors encouraged me, but the head nurse was hesitant.

"I've seen you walking a lot today already," she said. "You need to be in bed or sitting down to rest more. Your body is healing."

She promptly moved one of the red bucket chairs next to my bed and watched me as I walked over and sat down. No way was I going to cross her!

Sitting felt pretty good, except that the chair was very hard. I only had one pillow, so I couldn't really cushion myself a lot, but my body appreciated being in another position other than lying down. My abdomen was still incredibly sore and most movement was painful. I couldn't even turn over in bed without major reverse pressure and I could only lie on my right side for short periods of time because of the pain. It was also painful to sit upright after just a little while. It was as if my midsection couldn't fully support me. Then, I realized that sitting upright could be another step in my recovery. So, I added sitting in the chair to my regular routine of getting out of bed. I could walk *and* sit in a chair. Wow.

I've been privileged to participate in some awesome athletic challenges—district tennis championships in high school, swimming one mile a day during high school summers and in college, equestrian jumping routines, basketball, long-distance hiking, climbing up mountains—but walking around the ward and sitting up in a chair under my own power felt like I'd won some kind of championship. Thinking about it still makes me smile.

Dr. Theodore came in to check on my progress. He seemed impressed with how well my recovery was going. I was walking around, I could sit up without help (it wasn't pretty, but I could do it), and my digestive tract was working. With those milestones achieved, he cleared me to start drinking water. I was still on an IV, but he said I should try water and see how it went. I continued to run a fever of unknown origin and he didn't want to change anything more until they knew what was going on.

I was excited about water and sitting up and texted Jon. The kids nicknamed me "Aqua-Mom" when they were small because I was so insistent on everybody drinking plenty of water. I knew he'd know how much being able to drink water would mean to me.

———

Life in the ward once again became routine. My rash continued to come and go, but I didn't detect any pattern to it. I was also starting to feel like I was breathing through a mask. I could breathe fine, but my lungs felt like they were filled with fluid. Since I suffer from seasonal hay fever and it felt similar, I didn't really think anything about it. I figured that it was residual from the surgery or a byproduct of living in the public conditions I was in and breathing the unfiltered air coming in from the outside. Occasionally, I had trouble catching my breath, but again, I dismissed this as part of my recovery.

My mind continued to race. I was very aware of my surroundings, but I was having trouble calming my mind. It felt as if my brain was a spinning color wheel. Sleep was a refuge. I was exhausted and slept as much as possible, but in short bursts. I could shut out the noise of the ward, but the nurses were checking on me constantly and insisted that I respond to them. Looking back on it, I think they were checking on my mental acuity. I always made sure to pay close attention to them and do everything they said. I really didn't want to do anything that would signal that I wasn't on the road to recovery.

Jon was establishing a bit of a routine himself now that he was staying in Roseau.

From Jon:

"Wednesday was a relatively good day. I was able to get some much-needed sleep and I think Susan did too (all things considered). She texted me in the morning asking me to bring her a few things. While I was eating breakfast at the hotel I noticed a woman a couple of tables down with her arm in a sling. As I was leaving breakfast I ran in to the man who had been sitting with her. I asked if that was his wife and what had happened to her arm. He said that it was, and she had slipped at one of the waterfalls and broke it. They were from Germany and were wondering if they would still be able to make their flight on Friday. He asked where I was from and how long I was there for. I told him what had happened and he was very sympathetic. He said that a broken arm didn't seem quite that bad after hearing what happened to Susan.

"After breakfast I went to the small grocery store that was down the road from the hotel. I picked up a few things for Susan and headed back to the hospital. We were now regulars there, so I just walked right through (not that there was any security along the way anyway). Susan looked better than the day before. She was healing well and she seemed more alert. She was developing a rash on her arms and legs, though. We attributed it to the soap or something in the linens. At times it would also appear on her face and neck.

"We pretty much just hung out all that day in the ward. It was still a shock to the senses to be there and conditions were not good, but it's what we had to work with. We did some head shaking but we also realized this could easily have had a tragic ending. At one point during the morning we took inventory of the things we were grateful for. I remember saying to her that through this entire ordeal I never once felt that we weren't cared for by everyone who had helped us along the way. It was hard for me to say without crying. The impact of everything that had happened was starting to hit me now that I knew she was going to be okay and I could come down off autopilot a bit.

"Susan slept a lot that day. I walked around the area and did some things on my phone to keep in touch with the kids and my mom. We were all starting to feel like things were going to be okay."

I heard from my mom, who was starting to send me "get well" texts with news of her day. I appreciated getting these because it reminded me that life was normal somewhere. The kids kept up their texts to try to keep my spirits up. I was getting tired of being in the hospital and not feeling like my usual perky self. The kids had nicknamed me Suzy Sunshine when they were in middle school and still call me that today.

Katie: Hi mom! I'm thinking about you! I love you.

Me: Thanks, Mun. Not feeling like Suzy Sunshine today. Dad has update but all good. Just. Want. To. Come. Home.

Katie: I know, momma. You don't always have to be Suzy Sunshine. You are SO CLOSE!!! Do you have headphones? I'm sending every positive ounce of energy I have to you.

Me: I do and I know you are. This sucks more than you can imagine. Just trying to hang on a little longer. I can feel your love and concern. I couldn't do this without you, that's for sure.

Katie: I know it sucks. It would suck if you were going through it here too, just not as much. It's just one more day. ONE day. Just get through hour by hour and listen to all your favorite songs.

Me: Thanks. I did feel a hug in bed this morning when I was at a particular low point.

Katie: This always makes me smile. Love you.

Despite being in the middle of his clinicals as a physician assistant, Jimmy checked in regularly, too. He was trying to reassure me that my next procedure—to remove the drain the surgeon had left in—would be easier on me than my original surgery.

Jimmy: How are you feeling?

Me: Pretty good. Sore but not acute pain. A little nervous to have drain pulled tomorrow. Ready to go home.

Jimmy: Are u going under again for that?

Me: No clue.

Jimmy: It'll be ok. I've pulled drains out myself as a student. Don't sweat it. Keep thinking positive and moving forward so you can come home and relax.

Me: Thanks. That helps. Definitely moving forward.

Jimmy: Get some rest. We will check in again tomorrow. Love u.

Angels in Disguise

I received amazing care. The medical team had done everything in its power to save my life. There were no questions about race, nationality, or our ability to pay for treatment. I was simply a patient who needed their expert care. Long after I'd returned stateside and recovered fully, a friend said that she was sure that my treatment was special in some way. She was convinced that from the moment I stepped into the hospital, everyone knew I was an American citizen and that I should receive the best care possible. Neither Jon nor I believe that. From what we saw, everyone was treated with the same compassion and medical expertise. We were just patients, plain and simple.

"The nurses all took their jobs very seriously in a calm, assertive way," Jon said, "but most of all they really seemed to care about each patient. We had a lot of confidence in them, which made a huge difference for both of us."

I want to introduce you to my two ward neighbors. To my right was an elderly woman who wasn't doing well. She'd been hit by a car and was in critical condition. Her family kept a twenty-four-hour prayer vigil at her bedside and didn't expect her to live. She was mostly unconscious, but occasionally she would awaken crying. I overheard her family saying that she needed to stabilize before the doctors could fix her broken bones. Despite all of this, her family changed her sheets daily, bathed her, and made sure that she was well cared for. Her nurses also kept a close eye on her just as mine did for me. I didn't catch this woman's name, but when her family came in, I'd nod in sympathy for their situation.

The bed on my left had two patients during my stay. The first was a young woman of about thirty named Adrienne who had broken her arm. It hadn't healed properly, and she was in to have steel rods inserted to help with healing. I spent a lot of time talking with Adrienne, who was usually very happy and singing along with the Christian music that constantly played in the ward. She explained that she was the youngest of eight children (six brothers and one sister), all of whom still lived on the island. They lived in a village far from Roseau, but her brothers worked in the city. At least three of these men came in every day to visit her and pray with her. Her oldest brother usually came when Jon had stepped out to eat or to stretch his legs.

"How are you doing today?" Adrienne's older brother said in his Caribbean-accented English while he was waiting for her to come back from some tests.

"I'm fine," I said from my bed. I tried to smile, but it was obvious that I was in a lot of pain and not able to move very well.

"Do you mind if I pray for you?" he asked.

I nodded. I was unable to pray for myself. I just couldn't keep a focused thought in my head long enough to have any type of conversation with God about me, although I was able to pray for others—Jon, the kids, and the ladies in the ward.

"God of mercy and love, I ask your prayers for your servant Susan," he began as he bowed his head and gently raised his hands over me.

He never touched me, but I felt warmth rise up within the core of my broken body.

"Surround her with grace and heal her body and spirit so that she may continue to do your work," he continued.

I was humbled by this man's faith and grateful that he was led to share it with me. Once he finished, I felt calmer and very much surrounded by the presence of God.

When Jon was out on Wednesday afternoon, Adrienne's brother asked me if I wanted him to stay until Jon returned so I didn't have to be alone. Adrienne was visiting with other members of her family at that time and didn't need him. I was overwhelmed by this offer. I declined because I needed to get some sleep, but to have a complete stranger reach out to me to offer comfort and support was one of the kindest gestures I've ever experienced. Even in my confused mental state, I was able to recognize somewhere in the depths of my soul that Adrienne and her family were angels sent to reassure me in person that I was going to be okay.

The second patient to my left once Adrienne went home was a teenager who was in the hospital to have an abortion. I suspected this because she arrived after hours and her boyfriend and her mother stayed with her until her surgery. I didn't talk much to this family because they kept to themselves. The mother, who was genuinely concerned for her daughter, looked a little exasperated with the whole situation. The boyfriend seemed disconnected from everything and very uncomfortable in the women's ward. The young woman was both childlike and an adult at the same time. I felt very sad for the whole family because they were so disconnected from each other. I tried as best as I could to send positive energy their way for what I figured would be a long emotional recovery for all of them.

Another woman in the ward had had both legs amputated above her knees. She was several beds down from me, but I passed her as I was taking my walks and if she caught my eye, I made sure to smile and nod. She was usually alone, but she did have her own sheets and some personal items around her bed. I can't imagine what this woman had gone through. Every morning when the nurses changed her dressings, she would cry out in pain and ask God to show mercy on her. One particularly painful day, she begged the nurses to show her compassion and not change her dressings. They must have given her additional painkillers at that point, because her screams became whimpers as the nurses did their work. The nurses later walked by my bed carrying the used bandages to the medical disposal area. I offered prayers of healing and mercy as often as I could for this woman.

I would bring Jon up to speed on my neighbors in the ward when he came in, and I shared with him the story of my sandals and the warning from one of the other ladies in the ward. It was a good lesson for both of us to see past the window dressing to the authenticity of the people.

I tolerated drinking the bottled water and was getting stronger. I still had to take a nap after each five-minute spot of walking or sitting in the red chair, and every movement was painful; but I was getting the hang of being in the hospital. This stay in Dominica was the longest I'd ever spent in a hospital before. Despite how bad I felt, I was getting a little restless and really wanted to go home. Dr. Theodore had come back to check on me and said that if my fever would break, then he would take out the drain the next day (Thursday). I was ecstatic! This would put me one step closer to getting out of the hospital and heading home! The nurses started to give me some pills by mouth in addition to the many drugs still being given through my IV to try to help my fever go away.

———

Jon left the hospital about 4:30 that afternoon to miss all the crazy traffic on the way back to the hotel. While he was gone, I took another nap and settled in for the evening. Part of me was sad that he was leaving, but I also insisted that he go. There wasn't anything he could do for me and I could tell that the chaos of the ward was starting to get to him. I knew it would only be a matter of time before his anxiety stressed me out.

Don't get me wrong here . . . Jon was amazing throughout this whole ordeal. He was with me every step of the way and fully put my needs ahead of his own. That said, caregiving is often the hardest job when a loved one is sick. It's definitely one of the most thankless. Jon needed some time outside in fresh air away from the hospital. He also needed to be surrounded by people who weren't sick. I'd been worried all along that he was so alone. I had an entire medical team looking after me and now a tribe of women watching over my every move. He had no one, or so I thought.

"I went to the store and bought some beer," said Jon. "I went back to the hotel. There was a little porch in front of the room, so I sat there for an hour or so and had a few beers. While I was there every single person I had met the night before and that morning stopped by to see me and ask about Susan. The manager of the hotel met me when I drove in, the German couple stopped over to ask about her, the young man I'd met stopped to ask about her, and the bartender made a special trip over to ask about Susan. They were truly concerned and cared about her and us. It was a nice feeling knowing that so many people who were basically strangers showed such genuine concern for us."

Jon texted me before he went to bed.

Jon: All of the people I met last night and this morning have all made a point to approach me and ask how you are doing. I'm sitting outside my room having a beer and they all came to see me. You're famous.

Me: Very nice of them. Glad you landed in a supportive spot. Three of Adrienne's brothers are here and the one you met asked after you and if you needed anything. He even offered to do a food run!

Jon: Can't say a bad thing about anyone we have met here.

Me: Ditto

Jon: Can you let me know if they tell you what time they expect to take your tube out tomorrow?

Me: I will. I understood that the doctor would do it when he checks me in the early AM.

Jon: Ok. I don't think I'll be there by then. Meem asked if I took any crosses on the trip. I told her I did although I wasn't sure why when I packed them. Good ol Meem.

A few years ago, Jon started making comfort crosses. Some people call them clutch crosses or crisis crosses. They're wooden crosses that are designed to fit in the palm of your hand. Many people hold them close when they pray. Jon's are made from wood from our property. We also have some from trees that were felled by his dad and from furnishings in the original farmstead that his mother grew up on. Jon has felt called to give these away at random. I've done the same. We also started a family tradition at Christmas. We give one cross to each of the kids (all four—we consider our children by birth and their spouses all *our kids*) with the stipulation that they give it away to someone who they think needs it. Then, they report back to the family their story. These random acts of service have been a blessing to all of us.

I always keep a cross with me. Jon, as he noted, had brought some extra crosses with him to Dominica. We continued our late-night texting.

Me: I want to give a cross to Adrienne when she leaves (she's hoping tomorrow). Her family has been amazing. Do you have one I can use? This one has really helped me a lot.

Jon: I brought two. Yes, please give one to whoever you feel the need. That's why I packed them. I was going to suggest you give that one away anyway.

Me: Thanks. LU *(our code for Love You)*

Jon: Funny how something special comes from near tragedy. I'm guessing she'll be very touched.

Me: I hope so. Her big brother said he could tell that *I'm a woman of God*. Wasn't that nice?

Jon: It was. They both seem very genuine.

Me: I'm still thinking this is a story worth telling. Lots of eye-opening angles. Could be very inspirational.

Jon: Agree

Me: We could write it together

Jon: So many people involved. Some with more parts than others but as I think about it, all the pieces fall in to place.

Me: I have lots of things to put in. All angels in disguise. This all happened for a reason. Even the things we did before we left home.

At this point in my recovery, I was able to keep up with texts and short conversations pretty well. My breathing still felt strange and my chest was now feeling like I couldn't take a full deep breath. It felt like I had a bad chest cold except that there wasn't any mucus to cough out and I was wheezing some. Since the nurses were checking my vitals every hour on the hour and hadn't said anything about my lungs being filled with fluid, I assumed that I was fine and disregarded the breathing symptoms.

My mind was still on high alert to my surroundings and to my health in order to be an advocate for my care. Even though I trusted the nurses and doctors completely, I had an uneasy feeling. I just couldn't shake the sensation that I wasn't fully engaged with the world and that something wasn't right. The rash and fever continued and no one knew why. It was all a little unsettling.

Moments of Grace

I didn't get much sleep on Wednesday night. There was a lot of activity in the ward that evening. Adrienne had her usual gang of visitors and the family of the accident victim was continuing to keep a prayer vigil. In addition, the ward was overflowing with people. All the beds were full and just about everyone had at least two visitors. It was noisy and hot. I was restless from being confined to either the bed or the chair for so long. I couldn't walk around the ward because there were so many people. And, I was starting to become unfocused again. The rash was itchy and wouldn't go away. My insides felt like they were getting twisted around, as if my organs were trying to move back into their rightful places within my abdomen, which hurt a lot. The nurses were becoming even more obsessed with my fever and checking me about every half hour.

I tried to sleep but only dozed. My ability to tune out the world around me wasn't working its usual magic. I was tired and having a hard time calming myself down. My mind started racing again. I attempted reading but couldn't make sense of the letters on the page. I decided I needed some kind of mantra to focus on.

I took a deep cleansing breath. And another. And another. I didn't feel my usual sense of calm. I was starting to freak myself out a little. I almost texted Jon and the kids, but I didn't want to worry them. There wasn't much they could do. Besides, I knew that ultimately, I needed to take charge of my own recovery. I felt like I had poison inside me. I couldn't put my finger on it at the time, but I just sensed that something wasn't right. I didn't see the blackness I'd seen before, but I wasn't myself either.

I took another breath, but this time I said a simple mantra—"In with the good, out with the bad"—with each inhalation and exhalation. I tried hard to imagine myself breathing in a positive life force and breathing out all the bad vibes within me. I had to really focus on this with deliberate intent because I was so distracted and so disconnected from myself. It worked to steady me enough that I fell asleep in the early evening.

After a short while, my nurse came in to check on me. I'd only been asleep for about an hour or so. She was young and when I asked her how long she'd been a nurse while making small talk with her, she proudly told me that she'd been an RN for only one year. This put her at about age twenty-three or twenty-four in my book. She was highly professional and very sharp. She saw my rash, noted it, and then gave me some pills to help reduce my fever, which had spiked to a little over one hundred degrees. I was afraid that the rising fever would prompt some other kind of treatment and I just couldn't handle anything else.

Just when I thought I was going to spiral downward into a medical abyss, my nurse brought me screeching back to reality. She spotted my iPhone in its purple case. She looked around quickly, saw that the head nurse wasn't in sight, and shyly asked me if she could ask me a personal question. I agreed immediately, and she started asking me about my phone, my apps, and how I liked it.

She said that while cell phones were the norm for phone service on the island, they didn't always get the latest technologies quickly. She was curious about my phone because she'd read about it. I handed it over to her to look at and she enjoyed a few moments checking it out. You could have knocked me over with a feather. Here I'd been thinking of her and her colleagues as medical professionals only and not as people. I was grateful in that moment to be reminded of the world outside the hospital just when I needed to be able to talk about something other than my medical situation.

I felt a little calmer after our conversation. My mind was still racing, but a little slower than before. I still concentrated on slowing myself down with my breathing mantra, but I really felt that the universe had conspired to bring some simple humanity to me at just the right time. I lay in bed smiling over our conversation.

About 10:00 p.m., the head nurse kicked everyone out of the ward. Visiting hours were over and she wanted to quiet things down so patients could sleep. Also, a bunch of new patients were coming in and all beds were already full. The nurses were starting to put beds in the middle of the aisleway until they could figure out what to do with everyone. The commotion woke me up. Plus, I needed to use the bathroom and walk around now that the pathway was clearing.

I rolled myself out of bed, clutching my abdomen as I stood, then pushed my IV pole to the bathroom. By this time, I knew the drill and had my own stash of toilet paper and a towel to dry off with after washing my hands. I pulled out the metal bedpan, balanced it on the toilet, and took care of business. I was still limited to drinking bottled water, but my system had tolerated it pretty well, so I wasn't in the bathroom long. I decided to take one more walk around the ward. On my second pass down the long aisleway, the head nurse told me I needed to go to bed and try to get some sleep.

I hurt all over. My hips were developing bursitis from the weird sleeping and sitting positions I had to maintain in order to minimize my pain and not disrupt my IV. My IV had blown out of one hand and had to be repositioned in the other one. My skin was getting slimy and sticky because I couldn't take a shower due to the drain and the stitches. I did my best to wipe down with soap and water, but my rash was painful. I tried to wash myself off with some facial cleansing wipes I'd brought, and they helped a little. I clung to the idea that I'd be getting my drain out the next day and got back into bed.

In the middle of the night I awoke to shouting between the nurses and people outside the ward who wanted to get in. The shouting was highly unusual, as the nurses were strict about keeping the ward as calm as possible. I'd never heard them raise their voices to anyone, even patients who were less than gracious and shouting insults at them during painful treatments. Even when the ward was full of people, the general tone was more hushed than not. I hadn't been asleep long, but the TV was off and the ward was quiet except for the shouting.

I couldn't catch all the words, but suddenly I saw the nurses meet in the middle of the ward, agree to something, and then station themselves in various locations throughout the space. Their movements were purposeful as if they'd been rehearsed. The head nurse locked the doors to the ward, which were usually left wide open. Someone started pounding on the doors. Another nurse made a phone call and it sounded to me like she was requesting help. The others locked the other doors and circulated among the beds as if they were checking on patients. I became very unsettled.

In all the time we'd been in Dominica, this was the first time that I felt truly scared. I wanted Jon but didn't text him because I knew he'd freak out. I wanted to go home. I was worried that someone was going to get in and harm us in the ward. I'm a fighter and generally maintain good situational awareness to stay safe. In the dark of the night in a strange country and knowing I would be unable to do anything physical to protect myself, I felt vulnerable. My mental state was already questionable. My mind continued to have a hard time focusing and my insides felt like they were buzzing. Plus, I couldn't breathe very well.

I stayed in bed and stayed quiet. I clutched my phone in case I needed to use it. I turned over to my left side so that I had a fighting chance to get out of bed if I needed to. I repeated my breathing mantra. Then, I dozed.

The anxiety of the nurses was palpable, but they never left their posts. They never stopped taking care of patients. Two men who were dressed as if they were some type of security or law enforcement team eventually came by. The head nurse appeared to be briefing them on the situation. I don't know if the people trying to force their way in were still around, but the security folks stationed themselves near the main doors and remained there all night. I slept fitfully because I thought I needed to remain as alert as I could. At this point, my self-preservation instincts and hormones were running in high gear and on overtime.

I just wanted the night to end and the morning light to stream through the open-air ward. I never did learn what all the commotion was about. From my bed, the business of patient care continued as usual.

It was Thursday morning now and the doctors were supposed to remove the drainage tube with the intention of a Friday discharge from the hospital. This was a moment I'd been waiting for. Once the tube was out I could eat solid food. Also, it was one step closer to getting out and getting back home.

The kids sent me early morning texts to cheer me on for the drain removal.

Jimmy: Good luck today with the drain removal. You will do just fine, it's pretty quick. Keep your head up and keep moving forward. Please keep Katie and I posted on everything

Katie: Good luck, Mom! Love you

Later that morning Dr. Robert appeared at my bedside and reviewed my chart. Temperature: one hundred degrees. He consulted with Dr. Theodore then reported back to me. They had decided to leave the drain in at least one more day, he said. In that moment, time stopped. I was crushed. I felt like my body was betraying me big time and I was mad, sad, and frustrated. I was sick and tired of being sick and tired and I just wanted to cry. I could feel my shoulders slump and my face drop. There were simply no words.

The doctor said he would adjust the drain but that it had to stay in. He was hoping to pull it out on Friday and discharge me then, but Jon and I weren't feeling very confident about this. Besides the stubborn fever, my rash was getting worse. I was practically inconsolable. It was such a letdown. I felt like the last little bit of light within me was now just a glowing ember struggling to stay lit rather than a bright flame. I texted Jon with the news. His feelings mirrored my own. We were both D-O-N-E.

Me: Nurse just took my temp. It's 100. Ugh. She gave me some aspirin thing. They aren't taking out the drain because of the fever.

Jon: I don't even know how to respond. I feel so bad for you.

Me: Two words ... air ambulance ... if they won't release me. I trust them. They saved my life. I just can't do this anymore. I know they want what's best for me. I'm just done. I want to cry.

Jon: I am.

Me: I'm close to it myself.

Jon: If the doctor won't release you tomorrow maybe ask him about that option. They would still need to be part of the process I'm assuming.

Me: I will and I think so too. Can you check out the site? Just in case!

Jon: I'll look.

Me: Trying hard to sit tight. I believe that my soul signed up for this but enough is enough! Maybe I can save something for my next life?

Jon: Just be honest with the doctor in the morning about your tolerance level. It's getting to the point of impeding your recovery. That's assuming he won't release you.

Me: Ok. Good point.

Jon: If he says he will definitely release you on Saturday how would you feel?

Me: I'll have to think about it. Not able to be rational right now. Too sad. I do trust him. I just want OUT.

Jon: You're also operating on very little sleep too, which isn't helping.

Me: I know but it's reality. Thanks for hanging with me and pulling me back from the ledge

Jon: We can't both go off together

Me: Just heard the brother of the woman in the next bed praying for her. Gave him a cross. He asked your name and I said Jon and that I hoped it brought his sister peace. We prayed for her recovery. I also gave Adrienne a cross and she seemed truly touched by it.

After I'd accepted the fact that I wasn't getting the drain out, I tried to rally a little. I was very focused on getting out of the hospital the next day if the fever would go away. I wanted out. I was cleared to eat solid food, but my first meal left something to be desired. After an IV diet for the better part of a week, I was afraid of putting anything in my body other than water. I knew that the IV was coming out and that they'd never let me out if I wasn't eating, so I tried to do my best.

The hospital kitchen wasn't a standard foodservice kitchen like you'd see in the States. It looked more like a kitchen in someone's home. I'm not really sure where the food was prepared because the stove didn't look large enough to feed so many people. Three times a day a woman would come by with a cart that had different meals for different patients. I'm not sure what others were eating, but my meals were a little different than what I believe would have been served in the United States. The first morning, I had some very greasy eggs. Lunch was some bread and cheese. Dinner consisted of some kind of beans and rice with bits of meat. It was the best meal because it was the most flavorful. I couldn't eat a lot, but I did my best.

With the IV gone, I knew I needed to continue to drink as much water as I could hold to keep flushing out my system. Bottled water had to be brought in, as it wasn't standard issue in the hospital. Most patients were native Dominicans and could tolerate the tap water. I wasn't about to take any chances. I was hungry for bananas, oranges, and yogurt, but I was afraid to ask for them from the foodservice staff. They'd all been so kind to me. I didn't want to give the impression that I was ungrateful for their care. I looked around the ward and noticed that the other patients were receiving food from their visitors.

Once again, Jon came to my rescue.

Me: Doctor doing something to the drain but not removing it. I am still registering temp fluctuation between normal and 99.6. He did say the incision is healing nicely. Still on track for release tomorrow if I can keep the fevers at bay. I can begin solid food. Nothing spicy or carbonated.

Jon: Sorry about the rough night. Hopefully only one more. So would they take the tube out tomorrow or still today? Release on same day if tomorrow?

Me: I think tomorrow and yes, I think discharge same day. All depends on fevers

Jon: K

Me: I'm really trying hard to stay focused on the positive. No travel planning until I am officially told I'm discharged. No waiting period though once I'm released

Jon: Nope, no travel planning yet. Just mental planning so far. We'll have to see how things go. I'm going to send updates to the kids and your office and then head up.

Me: Ok. Can you tell work not to expect me next week at all until I get an all clear from a US doctor?

Jon: Yes

Me: Thanks. LU Also can you bring a bottled water?

Jon: Yes. LU

Me: Also can you bring some yogurt and a spoon? We can figure out other food later. Very greasy eggs they just gave me. Want to take it slow. Any yogurt flavor ok except prune.

Jon: Ok. There is a nice grocery close by here.

Jon's day was as rough as mine.

"Thursday was a tough day emotionally for both of us. I have never seen Susan so desperate, which only made things worse for me. The extended family had looked into an air ambulance to try to get her home sooner. It was nice of them, but it wasn't like we could just *spring* her from the hospital and tell them we were leaving. There was also the severity of her condition that needed to be taken into consideration. She still could barely walk. She wasn't getting bad treatment. It was actually very good. The question at this point was her comfort, which seemed to be adversely affecting her healing.

"I did a lot of pacing of the hospital grounds that day. It wasn't very big, so it didn't take long. When you went out the front door you could see over the Caribbean. The hospital sat up on a hill, so you could see a long way over the water. If you looked behind the hospital you could see up into the mountains that were covered in jungle. The island was very beautiful. I remember thinking that here I was on a warm, beautiful Caribbean island in February and I didn't care. My wife was hurting physically and emotionally and all I wanted to do was get her out of the hospital and make arrangements to get home. A few people made comments that it was nice I had a couple extra days in the sun, trying to make our situation seem lighter. I remember thinking how insensitive it was for them to say that.

"I could get up and move around but Susan was confined to the conditions and could not change a thing. The hot, noisy, crowded ward was taking a big emotional toll. She asked me to stay a little longer that day, which I did."

Jon and I both dreaded the thought of me not being released on Friday. It was depressing. I was trying hard to keep it together and not cry. I was exhausted and in pain. My mental state was getting more and more convoluted. I was having trouble keeping track of my conversations and sat and stared a lot. The blackness I'd experienced before was visible in my mind's eye at a distance again. I didn't feel pulled toward it; I just felt its presence, which made me even more uneasy.

I like to think that I can handle a lot of things, but I can honestly say that I was as close as I've ever come to a complete emotional breakdown. I'd been holding it together as much as I could because I didn't want to add to Jon's worries. I also was concerned that the doctors might try to give me drugs to help with depression and I didn't want that. The thought of having to stay another day longer was too much to think about. Later, Jon said that he didn't think I'd be released the next day either, but he didn't say anything to me at the time. I think he knew I wouldn't have been able to handle it.

One of the best things about our immediate and extended family is that we rally. I'd told the kids about the drain not being removed and they jumped in immediately to cheer me up. They knew how down I was and I think they sensed that I was on the verge of a total breakdown. My body was healing nicely in some ways but failing me in others. I felt like the blackness was trying to look more and more appealing to me, but I still refused to let it win. I do admit, though, that it was getting harder and harder to fight.

Deep within my soul, I knew that I'd seen the light. I knew I was going to get through this because I'd been told that before I ever even knew my diagnosis. Even with that knowledge, however, I let my humanity take over. I just didn't think I was up to the task of pushing forward any longer. The blackness looked increasingly inviting and definitely like the easier path. It would have been easy to surrender to it, but I just couldn't. There was something in me that simply refused to let the blackness win.

I tried to keep up a good front with the kids (always *The Mom*), but at this point I really needed to be more human with them and borrow some of their light. Their support made a huge difference on that very dark day. I needed them, they showed up, and I let them take care of me. I let their light surround me, support me, and protect me. It was then that I saw them as adults in their own right rather than as my adult children. I surrendered to their emotional support and tried to be present in the moment with them.

As parents, we're conditioned to love, protect, and serve our kids. It's instinctive and tribal for most of us. Being on the receiving end of that same love, protection, and service from our kids is humbling. It's hard. It's also one of the greatest joys imaginable. While I've always been proud of Katie and Jimmy for who they are and their unique gifts, I now saw them in a new way that made me even prouder. Also, I knew in that moment that if something happened to me, they'd be okay and be able to push forward. Not every parent has the privilege of seeing their kids in this way. I'm honored that the universe conspired to give me the opportunity to do so. Even now, when I think about what they did that day, I get teary-eyed. It was so full of unconditional and genuine love. It was true light.

Jimmy: Hey, Mom — We know you're getting anxious and ready to come home but trust the process and keep fighting this thing. It's not a step backwards by any means, it's just a different direction forward. We are all behind you on this. Don't forget that.

Katie: Yeah!! It's not a step backwards at all!

Me: Thanks, guys. I want to come home. I'm tired, the water makes me itch and it is hard to rest when there's 20+ other people in the ward plus relatives and medical personnel. Just at a low point today. Care has been excellent. I would rather be safe than sorry. This was too close of a call. Good news is that the doctor has been surprised at how fast my sutures etc. have healed which is good news. Also, the woman in the bed next to me said my surgeon is from her village and when she realized he was my doctor she was impressed. He has an excellent reputation. I've been very lucky along the way with many angels watching out for me. So has Dad. Thanks for keeping the family informed. Love getting texts from them. I'm just not up to jumping with both feet just yet. Onward!

Jimmy: Just get better. There's no rush. The fact that you're so anxious to get out of there shows you're improving...not having patience is your baseline and what you're known for ;) Keep that in mind but do not rush anything. We are all here waiting for ya and are not going anywhere.

Me: I know. Thanks! Just need some regular reminders today and tomorrow. Love you guys. Medical patience is definitely not my strong suit but all that has to change with this one. I've read that in the US recovery can be anywhere from 2 weeks – 3 months to get fully back for active people. Major wake-up call for me for sure.

Jimmy: Don't get caught up on the time frame for recovering right now. Work and everything else can wait. Just take it one day at a time, regardless of how slow it may seem.

Me: They just shortened the drain. Hoping the fever stays down. Any tips other than water which I'm setting records for? Mur ... doctor said drain as long as my arm. Said everything looks good. He had a student assist. She was nervous until I said you were finishing PA clinicals and told her she was doing fine. She smiled. Guys, thanks so much for everything. I couldn't do this without you. Major reality check for me. I need you more than ever!

Jimmy: I bet that made you feel good to make her smile!

Me: It did. She was nervous in front of her preceptor. Her hands were shaking.

Jimmy: I know the feeling all too well!!

Later that day the kids checked in on me again. I was tolerating the food and water pretty well at this point, but not eating a whole lot. Katie was especially concerned about my mental state and did her best to cheer me up by telling me my skin would look so amazing from all my sweating in the stuffy ward. Jimmy was running me through medical checklists to really understand how my recovery was going. I wasn't receiving pain shots any longer and had been switched to taking acetaminophen regularly. My fever was still registering 99.5 and the nurses and doctors were sticklers for a normal reading of 98.6. My legs were also getting a little puffy from being in bed so much. I was walking as often as possible but it was still far less than what my body was used to. The more I walked, the more the leg swelling seemed to go down—one more motivator for staying active.

The kids had been keeping the family up-to-date on all that was happening. I had heard from everyone on and off, but when the kids knew about my despair on Thursday, Katie put out an all call. Texts poured in from just about every single family member. It was such a gift. I'm the oldest in my family and have always been the head cheerleader and support person for everyone else. I wasn't used to being on the receiving end of such an outpouring of love and concern. It was humbling. It was kind. It got me through a very tough day.

Family: Hi Susan – gosh so sorry your appendix decided to burst in Dominica. So glad and thankful you are ok! Scary experience. I am sure you would love nothing more than to be home. Hang in there, stay strong, sure hoping you can get home soon. Get well!!

Family: Hi Aunt Susan— my mom told me about what happened and that you are not feeling great. I am so sorry that happened to you and am sending you lots of love and positive thoughts. You are such a light to our family and I always feel so loved and valued by you. We all love you so much and you always help us to remember what is really important in life and are such a great adult mentor and role model for me. I hope you start feeling better soon, get some rest and be good to yourself. Love you!!

Family: Just wanted to make sure you knew I was here for you. Always thinking about you, bringing you some sunshine from my heart to yours. Love you!

Family: I hope things are improving and you will be able to return stateside soon. I've been thinking about you and praying every day for you to get well. It has been quite an experience for you to say the least. I'm thinking you may have a cool scar after all this. I love you very much and we are all keeping track of Jimmy and Katie. You have wonderful children and I'm proud to be their uncle.

A good friend of mine has a hilarious cat. She started sending me texts and "selfies" from her cat. It was just the kind of silliness I needed and made me smile.

My boss was checking in regularly by email with Jon, and I knew that everyone at work was really concerned, sending good vibes, and praying for my recovery. They offered incredible support at every turn, but Jon held them off until we got back to the US when we both knew we'd need some help. It was clear that I wasn't going to recover quickly from this ordeal.

Katie and Jimmy were working overtime to keep Jon's spirits up with phone calls and texts.

Jon: Tough day for her emotionally. She still registers a slight fever and she's afraid they won't let her go tomorrow. Won't be a good day if that happens.

Katie: They might let her go once they see how she reacts to them saying *no* haha.

Jon: Good point. I would expect her to break down. She's close now.

Katie: I'm coming to your house to take care of Mom and give you a huge huge HUGE hug and let you get in the woods, or whatever your heart desires. Me and Mema have got you covered.

Jon: Thank you, Litto! This has been very draining for both of us. You have been soooo helpful.

Katie: I'm glad I could be. I felt so helpless

Jon: I'm sure you did. I did too. But I was unable to do what you helped with. May have seemed small to you but it was great having someone at the command post.

Katie: We're a good team, Pod!

Jon: Yep!

Jimmy: NP. How's the day going for you guys?

Jon: Pretty good. Mom is "coming back." She is getting feisty and impatient, which I take as a good sign. Even if they let her out on Friday, travel will still be a challenge. She is obviously very sore.

Jimmy: I'm sure you're both getting a little bored and ready to head home.

Jon: Yes but also came to the realization earlier today that we were/are very lucky. This could have been tragic even if we were home. Everyone here has been awesome toward us. At no time have we ever felt that we haven't been cared for by anyone here.

Jimmy: It absolutely could have been. It scared the crap out of me. I don't think I'll be 100% anxiety free until you guys get home and settled for a few days. I feel some guilt too from not recognizing what was happening sooner than I did, despite it being via text. Good that the staff there is as good as they are, though. I hate to admit that I anticipated the worst, but it sounds like it has been much different.

Jon: How could you possibly have known? Even the doctors here couldn't be sure until they did a scan. I also anticipated the worst but we have been pleasantly surprised. Besides the facilities being below what we snobby Americans would consider standard, they have been great.

Whenever I hear of others going through something tough, I add them to my prayer chain. I also try to imagine them bathed in light and joy. I've never known if they feel a difference, but it's always made me feel good to try to ease their burden by connecting with them through the universe. As a survivor of a traumatic and dramatic health scare, I can say with conviction that I literally felt the love and good wishes of every single person who thought of me whether I knew them personally or not. It was like getting a big hug every day.

It's hard to explain, but in the midst of my own physical and emotional pain, I thought I was in a spiritual void. Boy, was I mistaken. I might not have been able to pray for myself, but hundreds of others took on that burden on my behalf. After I'd recovered, I was sharing my story with a good friend who said that he'd had a feeling that someone in his inner circle was struggling with something, but he couldn't put his finger on it. Being a highly spiritual person, he just put good vibes out to the universe and hoped that they reached the right target. His vibes and those of countless others absolutely did.

I am convinced that their love held me in the light even when I couldn't see it. It kept me sane. It gave me strength. It gave me patience. It made me smile. It guarded my spirit like a team of angels circling me with shields raised. It kept the blackness at bay. It was as real to me as the out-of-body experience I'd had in our cottage. And, it enabled me to endure the disappointment of Thursday and the dramas to come.

During that very down day, I experienced two moments of grace in the ward. First, I gave a cross to Adrienne. I told her that just as Dominica is a rare habitat, we lived in one, too, in Ohio, and Jon had made the cross from one of our trees. She was touched and I thanked her for being a nice friend during a tough time. Then I gave a cross to the family of the woman on my right. She wasn't doing very well. I told the woman's brother that I hoped it would bring her (and them) some peace. He smiled. I shared these stories with the kids over text and told them I was trying hard to stay focused on these moments of grace and be grateful that I was alive.

Katie and Jimmy wrote back after they heard the stories, as did my son-in-law, Mike, and my daughter-in-law, Megan, which was wonderful. The M-Squad (our family nickname for all four kids—Mun, Mike, Mur, and Megan) was continuing to show their love and support.

Jimmy: I figured you guys would have some crosses with you. Was only a matter of time before you gave them away at that place. We have all been thinking about you and cannot imagine a world without you in it. Keep getting better so you can come home ASAP.

Katie: The true sign of a strong and good-hearted person: being in a horrible situation and making OTHER people happy despite how miserable you are feeling. When Mema told me that you guys took 2 crosses with you, I knew it was meant to be for a good reason. They are lucky recipients to not only have received the crosses but to have met you guys too. There's a special place in Heaven for you and I'm beyond thankful that you didn't see it yet. You still have 46.5 years until your goal of being 100! I love you.

Megan: I'm glad that you were able to spread some faith and positivity to them. I can't imagine having to go through what you have this week. Stay strong, you will be home soon!

Mike: The human spirit is so powerful. It is amazing what we can do. Beautiful story, Susan. I'm sure your new friends appreciate your thoughtfulness and generosity. We are so happy that you are feeling better and so glad you are going home. Love you.

I had the unexpected pleasure of speaking with one of the medical students from the Ross Medical School, which was next to the hospital. Dr. Robert had brought over a class of students and they were practicing their patient interviewing skills. Since I was the only foreigner in the ward, he thought it might be good for one of his students to practice on me.

I've always been a huge supporter of any kind of practical experience in education and was more than happy to help. It broke up the monotony of the day. Also, the chance to focus on someone else's needs was a great redirect for my depressed mind.

My student was from India and had been raised in the United States. She spoke British English but was very familiar with American culture and seemed excited to have an American patient assigned to her. We made small talk, but she kept it very professional since her instructor was floating in the ward and dropping in to observe all patient examinations. She proceeded to examine me by taking my vitals and then interviewed me to learn about my story. I was able to sit up in bed and dangle my legs over the side, which gave her room to put her equipment on my bed. She did a great job and was very thorough. I kept thinking about my son doing similar kinds of things during his training to be a physician assistant and tried my best to help all that I could. It was a bright spot in the day.

Dr. Robert came up to me afterward to thank me. He told me that he was especially glad that his students had a chance to meet me. He said my case was a little unusual and my status as an American tourist added a cultural twist to the conversation that most of his students didn't have a chance to experience while at Ross, even though most students come from places other than Dominica. It's funny, but during my conversation with my student, my mind was more focused and clearer than it had been all day. I still had trouble breathing, but I was able to stay engaged a little easier. I think the universe was conspiring to give me a glimmer of hope that I was on the mend.

Throughout this whole ordeal, Jon was trying so hard to stay positive and keep me upbeat. The true test of a life partner is when the "for better or worse" and "in sickness and in health" vows are challenged. It never occurred to me that he wouldn't show up for me and do everything within his power to keep me safe. And he did with every fiber of his being every minute of every day.

Me (to the kids): Dad's been a trooper. Thanks for supporting him too. He hates hospitals and the chaos of this more than I do, but he's hanging in. Kind of jealous he gets to go to a quiet, AC hotel room each night. This sucks.

Jimmy: I talked to him yesterday for about two hrs about anything and everything and he seems like he is doing better. We just want u better and home, bottom line. I'm sure you are both incredibly burnt out and restless by now.

Me: Understatement of the day. I love the Caribbean, but we've put a minimum of a two-year moratorium on any travel south of the border.

Jimmy: LOL. Probably a good idea ;) Most people leave part of their heart in a place they love. A guess an appendix can work too.

"I felt bad leaving her that evening," Jon said. "Again, I could go back to my comfortable hotel room, but she was stuck. When I got back to the hotel I went and sat at a table near the water by myself. I didn't feel like sitting at the bar or socializing with anyone. I wanted to go home and I wanted Susan to be able to leave the hospital. She still had a lot of healing to do but I didn't think she could do that in the hospital. I ate and walked back to the room. The bartender stopped me on the way back to ask about Susan and to say hi. He was really a very nice guy and I felt like he really cared about us.

"There was a lot of texting from Susan that evening. I could tell she was scared, miserable, and increasingly desperate. The texts continued into the night as I was trying to go to sleep. At one point I sent her a pretty stern one that said basically *get a grip*. I felt bad sending it. Easy for me to say while I was in my private room with AC. She later said it was helpful even though it made her mad at the time. The kids sent her emails and texts too, telling her how much they loved her and knew she would be home soon. She said they read those throughout the night."

Jon: One last piece of tough love. This isn't going to change just because you want it to. The best thing you can do tonight is surrender to it. Worry about what happens next when he [the doctor] is there tomorrow. Getting all worked up about what might happen is not helping. I know I'm not living what you are and it looks like pure Hell but what other choice do you have?

Me: You're right. This is hard, but I guess isn't meant to be easy, is it?

Jon: Nothing easy about almost losing your life in a foreign country. While you are working on surrendering to a higher power you can also imagine a light entering the top of your head or base of your skull. It's probably purple, since that's what your color is. It slowly makes its way down each part of your body illuminating and healing all your cells. It is most bright in the areas that need the most healing. It is the light of all that is and is the source of your healing. It is also the light of pure Divine love. Try that. I have before and it seems to work. It's real!

Another Scare

I tried Jon's meditation and drifted off to sleep. I got up once to use the bathroom and didn't feel quite right. I was a little disoriented and dizzy. I figured that I hadn't had enough to drink that day, so I doubled up on water. While I was washing my hands, a fellow patient in the ward started talking to me. Her name was Tatiana. We each shared our stories.

"How are you?" Tatiana asked.

"I'm fine," I answered. "I'm feeling better every day, but I still can't leave."

"Where are you from?" she asked.

"The United States," I said. She smiled at that, but I wasn't sure what that meant. "How are you doing? Will you be here long?"

"I'm lucky," Tatiana said. "I came in here to have a growth checked. I just learned that it isn't anything to worry about. It was caused by an allergic reaction. I'm getting out of here tomorrow."

The conversation was so normal. I could have been talking to a friend or colleague. I had to work really hard to stay focused on what we were saying, and the room seemed to be on a slant to me; but I didn't really think that was out of the ordinary. Thankfully both our stories had happy endings: we were alive.

I shuffled back to bed. I was free of the IV pole, so maneuvering around the ward was a lot easier, but my abdomen was still in a lot of pain and I took very small steps while holding my abdomen protectively. I was having a hard time standing straight up, which I thought was a little weird but disregarded. I was physically exhausted from my surgery, recovery, and lack of sound sleep. I was emotionally a basket case. I could feel my brain getting hazy again and I felt kind of nervy and startled easily.

I went back to bed and fell into a deep, deep sleep—probably the deepest I'd had all week that wasn't medically induced. Then, in the middle of the night I woke suddenly, covered in sweat and breathing as if my lungs weren't working. My breaths were short and I was having a hard time filling and clearing them. I knew I wasn't at home but wasn't sure where I was. I was completely disoriented for a few long seconds.

I rolled myself up so I was sitting on the edge of my bed. I knew I needed to use the bathroom and struggled to get up. When the soles of my feet touched the rough concrete floor, I remembered to put on my sandals. Then, I stood at the foot of my bed and forgot the way to the bathroom. It was a few feet away from me and I'd walked the path many times, but I couldn't connect the disjointed thoughts in my head to figure out what to do. My eyes were having trouble focusing and I was losing parts of my vision. I thought at the time that I might be getting a migraine.

I started walking away from my bed. It felt like I was walking kind of tilted or that the room was on a slant. My subconscious was leading me to the bathroom, but I didn't realize where I was until I got to the door at the toilet stall. I used the facilities (thankfully, I remembered how to do that on my own!) and went to wash my hands still having trouble focusing my vision. I glanced up at myself in the mirror and was shocked at the image looking back at me. My face was covered with hives. One of my eyes was nearly swollen shut. I looked like the character Violet in *Willy Wonka and the Chocolate Factory*, who eats too much food and turns into a blueberry, except that I was pinkish instead of blue. I knew I needed help and made my way to the nurses' station.

My nurse that night was the young woman who had looked at my iPhone. I was having trouble getting the words that I was trying to form in my head to come out of my mouth and when they did, I felt like I was hearing my voice through water.

"I think I need help," I said to the nurse while pointing to my face. "I can't focus and it's hard to breathe."

The room was beginning to spin, and I grabbed the edge of the nurses' station. I'm not sure what the look on my face was, but she immediately sprang into action by coming out from behind her desk.

"Let's get you back to bed and I'll get the doctor," she said gently as she guided me back.

I couldn't understand everything she said, but she helped me into bed. She even took off my sandals and slipped them under my bed for me.

All of a sudden she put her face directly in front of mine and said, "I think you're having an allergic reaction." She explained she needed to get the doctor and some medicine. I was becoming more and more disoriented and I was really scared, even more than I had been when I first went to the ER.

A million thoughts flashed through my mind in quick succession. It was as if someone was flipping a light switch on and off over and over and over again. What was happening to me? My nurse returned with the resident on duty, Dr. Jones. The doctor examined me and appeared to concur with whatever the nurse had told her and my chart showed. The nurse gave me two shots through the port which was still in my hand and both of them stood hyperfocused on me.

Within seconds my breathing became more regular (or as regularly irregular as it had been before this incident), the flashes of light in my brain stopped, and the swelling from my hives started to go down. I could feel my eye opening slightly. Dr. Jones and my nurse were visibly relieved. The nurse helped me to drink some water and gave me some more medicine. The doctor was adamant that they needed to get to the bottom of the reaction but felt confident that it was one of the many antibiotics I was on. Unfortunately, the only way they could figure it out was through the process of elimination. In short, they were going to give me one drug at a time every thirty minutes and see what happened. They assured me that they'd have countermeasures in place to handle the allergic reaction when it came up.

Even in my confused state, I didn't think this was such a great idea. I was scared stiff about becoming so disoriented again. I knew I wouldn't be able to handle much more. My nerves were shot. Also, once I regained my wits I realized that if this couldn't be brought under control, it might prevent me from getting my drain pulled out the next day or, worst-case scenario, delay my release. I'd read that the typical recovery period for a ruptured appendix was four to six weeks, and in my confused state, all I could think was that there was no way I wanted to spend all that time in Dominica in bed number three of the Dawbiney Women's Ward, no matter how nice they were to me.

My nurse confirmed with me that I approved of the treatment recommendation. What choice did I have? It was late, but I texted Jon because I wasn't sure how this would end and I wanted him to hear from me what was going on.

I had one more allergic reaction during the trial-and-error process, but luckily the eagle eyes of the nurse caught it immediately and she was able to treat me. I didn't text Jon about the second one. One of us needed to get some sleep on the off chance that I'd be released the next day, although that was looking less and less like an option.

Turns out that I was allergic to one of the superdrug antibiotics they were giving me constantly. The rash came and went but wasn't necessarily linked to the times that the drug was given to me. I'm not sure if it built up in my system over time and caused the acute reaction or what happened. I didn't ask. I just knew that the rash covering my body was going away and that I was returning to some sort of new normal.

I texted Jon the next morning. It had become my habit to text when I woke up to let him know I'd made it through the night. The day before, we'd gotten in trouble for not paying for my medicine each day. In Dominica a lot of health care is free, but medicine isn't. We didn't know this. The head nurse on day shift had told me that I was racking up some big pharmacy bills by Dominican standards (a couple hundred US dollars—the same drugs would have been several thousand dollars in the States). I was embarrassed and apologized for not knowing the payment rules. I didn't have a way to pay the hospital and told her Jon would settle up as soon as he arrived for the day. With this latest incident, I knew we'd need to pay up again.

I also texted the kids, who by this time were keeping very close tabs on me. They were sending their good wishes for the drain to be removed.

Jimmy: What's your temperature?

Katie: *Pounding fists on the table* Remove the tube! Remove the tube! Remove the tube!

Me: Thanks, Mun! Me too.

Jimmy: When's the next time the doctor is seeing you?

Me: Usually between 8-10 am. Updates ASAP. Full ward right now

Wow. I was starting to realize the many angels along the way who were watching out for me. If I'd been released earlier, the result could have been much more serious. With this rash taken care of, my skin was feeling a lot better. My mind was still a mess, though, and I found it hard to concentrate for very long. My medical team was aware of everything about me, but we agreed that it was best to give me the time, rest, and quiet I needed to heal. If I had pressed them, I believe they would have given me some medication to calm me, but I didn't want any more meds. The antibiotics were critical and doing their job (now that we'd eliminated the one I was allergic to). I really wanted to follow a more natural path toward healing. I was working my breathing mantra like crazy. It felt like it was the only thing that was keeping me sane (and even that was debatable at this point). I was exhausted and dozed until the shift change from night to day. And that's when I had a moment of clarity.

The head nurse was chastising my night nurse for not following the medicine request (i.e., procurement) protocols. From what I could tell, my nurse got the medicine from another department, which was located closer to my ward, because it was faster and she felt it medically necessary to have the drugs on hand due to the severity of my allergic reaction. The head nurse was professional and never raised her voice, but she was very stern. As soon as I realized what was going on, I started to sit up in my bed. My nurse—a woman with only one year of experience—figured out something that none of us had been able to figure out for close to a week. There was no way I was going to let her go down on my account.

I was under strict orders to stay in bed unless I had to use the restroom or until my doctors arrived. I managed to sit up against my pillow and the wall at the head of my bed. I continued to watch and listen to the nurses' conversation. My nurse listened intently and respectfully. She then acknowledged the protocol breach and held herself accountable to it. She also stood her ground very firmly on the medical rationale for her actions. There was silence. I saw them looking straight into each other's eyes. There were no arguments, just two colleagues trying to do their best. The head nurse then praised my nurse for her *smart problem solving* and said that there would be no official reprimand in my nurse's file.

I breathed a sigh of relief.

Freedom!

I figured the chances of release on Friday were slim to none with all the allergic reactions the night before. My surgical scars were healing nicely, I was tolerating food, I was fairly mobile (all things considered), and my vital signs other than the fever were very normal. My medical team, however, was incredibly cautious. I was trying to rally, with little success, for what I expected to be another long day in the ward.

I was focusing on my breathing mantra to try to bring some calmness to my mind. I wasn't experiencing the dizziness any longer, but I still had a hard time concentrating. My brain was just rapid firing sparks of light inside my head. It was like looking at the old-fashioned Tilt-a-Whirl ride at the county fair all lit up at night—spinning, spinning, spinning. I was working hard not to succumb to this whirlwind inside my brain and it was tough. I continued to experience some trouble breathing, but it was like the feeling I've had during a bad hay fever season. My lungs felt heavy as if they'd gained weight and my chest muscles weren't totally capable of supporting them. I also had to clear my throat often, which was kind of annoying. On the good side, I didn't feel the same problems I'd had the night before, which was a huge relief!

I started my day with my usual texts to Jon, then had a sponge bath. Since I hadn't been able to shower for nearly one week, I felt slimy and my hair hung in long, messy strands. I looked like I'd just camped out for a week and reemerged into the world—not pretty! Sponge baths just aren't the same as a hot shower.

By the time I was finished with my morning routine, the doctors had arrived in the ward and were making their rounds. I could see them talking with my nurses, but I wasn't sure if they were talking about me. I watched as my doctors circled the ward. Finally, they reached my bed. I was a little embarrassed about my hygiene, or lack thereof, but told myself that I wasn't the first patient not looking or smelling her best in this hospital. Also, my sheets, still the originals I received when I was first admitted, were going to need to be changed if I had to stay much longer. Dr. Theodore didn't seem to mind my circumstances at all. He examined me and we talked for a few minutes about how I was feeling. He remained very surprised and pleased about my recovery from the surgery.

"I heard you had some problems last night," Dr. Theodore said as he began to examine me. The young nurse who had treated me on the night shift was standing by to assist, if needed.

"I did, but everyone here took very good care of me," I said. "It seems the rash that kept coming and going was because of one of the drugs I was on. The resident and this nurse figured out what was going on and I feel a lot better."

Dr. Theodore and Dr. Robert, who was also standing by, nodded in agreement as I spoke. Clearly, they had already heard all the details and neither one seemed overly concerned. The rash was gone, and my eye and face were back to normal size. As usual, Dr. Theodore opened my bandaged side to examine my incision site. Suddenly, he smiled.

"I'm glad to hear that," he said. "Your fever is gone. We believe it was related to the allergic reaction, which we've taken care of. You're feeling fine, right?"

"Yes," I confirmed. "I'll have to add that drug to my list of allergies in case anyone else needs to know it in the future."

Dr. Theodore told me it would be in my hospital records and then gave me the best news I'd heard in a long time.

"This is really looking good," he said, gesturing to my incision site. "You've come a long way and I think we can take out the drain today. Dr. Robert will take care of that. Then, I think we can release you, with a few conditions."

I didn't think I'd heard him right. There had to be some kind of mistake. They were just messing with me. I looked at Dr. Theodore and said, "Really? You're letting me out?" He smiled broadly and said that if I promised to do exactly what he said, he'd release me.

I was getting out of the hospital!

Dr. Robert smiled and left to see to his next patient. Dr. Theodore laughed a little but quickly regained his extremely professional demeanor.

"Do you have a place to stay in Roseau?" he asked. "You have to stay in the city in case anything comes up. I also want you to share your travel plans with me. You'll need to check in with me at least once before you head home and I'll provide you with some medicine to make it easier to travel. I'm on call all weekend in the hospital so I'll be here and easy to reach. You can just come here, and I'll see you. You don't need to make an appointment."

He gave me his personal cell phone number and made me promise to contact him directly day or night with any questions or concerns. I was floored. In all my years as a patient I have never been given a direct line to a doctor. I was humbled by his willingness to see my care through all the way until I left for the States. I quickly agreed to all of Dr. Theodore's terms.

Nothing about my physical and mental situation had changed, but in that moment, I felt like I'd hit the jackpot of life. I knew I had a long road ahead of me and neither Jon nor I had any idea how we were going to get home, but I experienced a lightness of spirit that I don't remember feeling before. I didn't have to sleep in the ward again. I could sleep through the night. I could go outside and see the sun. I was euphoric!

My doctors conferred with each other again and set in motion all the things that had to happen for me to be released. It was the crack of dawn, but they seemed to think that I'd be released by lunch.

I was so relieved, I cried tears of joy silently in my bed. I couldn't believe it. I immediately texted Jon.

"When Susan texted that she was being released, I was prepared for the exact opposite news, so the instant relief quickly turned to emotion which turned to tears," Jon recalled. "She was getting out. She had made it over the biggest hurdle. Words can't describe the relief I felt. The doctor's conditions weren't a problem. Just let her out!"

Once Jon got to the hospital, there were more tears. We just clung to each other. By this time, we'd let the kids know.

Me: Doc releasing me today on condition I stay in Roseau tonight, call him with travel plans, see him once as outpatient and take medicine for travel. One happy girl here. Earliest travel would be Sunday/Monday. Dad in charge of logistics. Don't let up on prayers and good wishes. Too many weird things have happened. You guys are my lifeline right now!!! I love you!

Jimmy: That just made me tear up. Amazing news. Follow his orders and do not take them lightly. Thinking of you.

Me: Crying here too, there's a light at the end of the tunnel. Will follow all orders to the letter. I'm a changed woman on that

Jimmy: It was always there. Just not a linear path.

Katie: I burst into tears. Are you free yet!?

Me: Halfway there. Dad paying final bills and waiting for final discharge review and meds.

Jimmy: So happy you're leaving. Huge relief I'm sure for u. For Katie and I too.

Me: Thanks! No argument here. One more thing we're waiting for and then out.

Jimmy: My typical Friday night celebratory bourbon has a whole other meaning this week. Rest up this weekend!

Me: Will do! So grateful. There are no words.

Jimmy: Cheers to mom!!

Katie: Cheers! Got a Moscow mule on deck.

Me: Thanks, guys!

I've never been hospitalized for longer than two nights before and that was when I gave birth to our daughter, so the release was great news! Princess Margaret Hospital had been a safe haven for me for nearly a week. It was a lifeline—literally—during the most traumatic and dramatic time of my life. As I sat on the bed and looked around the ward at the nurses, the foodservice ladies, the cleaning team, the plumber who had finally come in to fix the broken toilets, and the other patients and their families, I was filled with such a sense of gratitude. This was no simple thank you. It started in the tips of my toes and filled me up to the top of my head. My heart was full and I was very emotional.

My body hurt, and my brain was still doing battle with itself, but my spirit was soaring. To this day, I recall the faces, the smiles, the compassion, and the expertise of the women and men whose only mission was to make sure that I healed. I didn't fit the typical Dominican profile. I could barely speak the language. I had a very biased view of what health care should look like. None of that mattered. I was just another soul who needed them. And they took me in no questions asked.

Jon and I agreed that we needed to hold it together until we got out of the hospital. We knew we had some serious processing to do, but we were both so completely drained that we tried our best to set the heavy stuff aside and focus on each of the many next steps ahead of us to get out of the hospital and off the island. We were ready to go home.

Jon had gone to pay all the bills. My brain remained foggy and while I was finishing more of my own sentences by this time than I had pretty much all week, I didn't trust myself to handle anything important other than signing myself out of the hospital.

By this time, we knew that our health care and trip insurance should cover most of the expenses. We had no idea what to expect for costs. The drug prices had been so much less than what we were used to, but this was a multinight hospital stay, complete with surgery, surgeon, other doctor fees, and more. Everyone had been so nice to us that we didn't want to subject the hospital or the doctors to the pain of navigating the US health insurance system. While our coverage was good, the paperwork was a burden on its best day and we just couldn't bring ourselves to inflict that on anyone. Luckily, we had some options.

From Jon:

"I figured we would be there all day waiting for the paperwork to be done so we could leave. The surgeon had asked to see me right away. I went down to where he was but he was not available, so I went back to the ward. We settled the bills for the medication Susan was given. That was all paid in cash for some reason, but okay. It was cheap.

"The surgeon called up and asked that I come back down again. He had a separate bill that he wanted to settle up. He wanted our US insurance information so he could file a claim. I told him that we could pay with a credit card and we would file with insurance if that would help him. He said that he wasn't sure if he could accept a card, but he would look into it. He said he would come and find me.

"A short time later someone from the billing department came to find me to settle the hospital bill. We went down to the accounting department, he had the bill, which was not very much, I gave him a credit card, done. After the card was run, I noticed he had billed something twice. He immediately reversed the original charge, adjusted it, and charged the correct one. All very easy.

"I went down to the outpatient area to wait for a bit. The surgeon saw me and called me in. He had found a way to accept a credit card. It must have been a friend of his or something. It was for a different business, so they must have worked something out. Regardless, I paid for the procedure—again, cheap—and everything was done. I walked back up to the ward to get Susan. We had packed up all her things earlier and were ready to go. We thanked the doctor and the nurses for everything they had done for us and began the slow walk to the front door. We were out of there by 12:30 p.m."

During this time, the head nurse came over with the discharge paperwork and drugs for me to take after discharge. The hospital also had a letter of certification for the procedure for our local doctor to keep on file. There were a couple of typos that needed to be corrected but they were taken care of within minutes. I was a little nervous about the idea of carrying drugs into the United States and I wanted all paperwork to be perfect. They were prescriptions and clearly labeled, but they were in small, plastic zipper bags. I didn't want anything to stand between me and entry back into the States.

The new American administration had enacted some stricter travel and customs rules during our stay in Dominica, which had been widely reported on the Christian TV station blaring all day. These new rules were the subject of a lot of conversation in the ward. Being the only American present, I chose to say nothing, but it pained me that this negativity was the impression that most were getting of America, especially when their country had welcomed Jon and me so warmly. I hoped that my own actions spoke better of America than what they witnessed on TV.

I hadn't been dressed in more than a hospital gown or a night-gown for close to a week. Jon had brought over my baggiest sports shorts, a ballcap to hide my very dirty hair, and one of his cotton shirts. I was able to dress myself, but it was painful. Putting on clothes requires a lot of twisting and turning that I'd forgotten about. My insides were still very painful and I had a big sterile bandage taped to the lower right quarter of my abdomen. The resident who taped me up put extra tape over the gauze on my incision site to keep everything as sterile as possible during our trip home. Dr. Theodore told me in no uncertain terms to keep the bandage dry and that I wasn't to remove the bandage until I got home, even though we didn't know our travel plans yet.

I later learned that I'd lost about twenty-five pounds in the hospital and many inches from my body. My clothes hung on me, but I didn't care. I was wearing clothes! I wasn't allowed to carry anything heavier than my sandals, so Jon carried my small bag in one hand and offered his other arm to me. I was going to walk out of the hospital on my own power (sort of)! At this point, every single step I took was still very painful. Instead of the charley horse I felt when my appendix was still inside me, it felt more like a major bruise. The surgeon had cut through every muscle in my abdomen and stitched up some of my internal organs. I still had a lot of healing to do.

I hadn't been outside of the ward for close to a week, the lone exception being when I'd been wheeled in to the operating theater from the emergency room. Walking out of the hospital was like walking into a whole new world for me. I started crying at the pure joy of being able to breathe fresh air. To feel the sun on my face and to see the beautiful flowers and trees of Dominica was such a gift. It was like I was seeing the world for the first time and it filled me with a sense of wonder at the sheer simplicity of being alive. I was so happy!

Getting into our little car was tricky for me. I'd been mostly lying down and walking for the past five days. The little sitting I did was still kind of stretched out and I couldn't sit for very long. I hadn't been crunched up like I'd need to be to sit in our car. We still had the same little RAV4 we'd used before I was sick and I more or less backed into my seat and swung my legs around to get them in. I couldn't put one foot in the car, balance, and then put the other in, as that would require too much twisting, and my core just didn't support me well. Besides, I wasn't strong enough to stand on one leg yet, particularly on my right side. I continued to apply reverse pressure to help ease the constant pain and protected my right side with my hands.

En route to the hotel, Jon drove through the botanical garden, which was quite lovely and kept us away from the crazy drivers in Roseau. The city was filling up because the festival of Carnival was about to start and lots of celebrations, including a major parade, were getting under way. I noticed everything! The children in their very colorful school uniforms. The different greens of the plants. The vibrancy of the flowers. A bunch of kids playing soccer. It was so renewing. I just felt like I had a chance to look at the world in a new way and I really liked it.

Once we got back onto the main thoroughfare, I felt every single bump in the road and the lack of shocks on the car. I adjusted my seat so I was leaning back a little to take some pressure off my abdomen and applied a lot of pressure underneath my seatbelt. I was focused on my breathing mantra to make sure that I could manage the pain.

When we reached the hotel, I followed Jon into the room that had been his home while I was in the ward. As we were walking, the owners told me that once they'd learned about our story from Hervé when the original reservation for Jon was made, they made sure to assign us a first-floor room so I could avoid stairs as much as possible. That kind gesture really touched my heart. They didn't even know us but took us in like family.

As for the room . . . It was air conditioned! There was a working toilet and not a bedpan in sight! It was quiet! I'd become so desensitized to the constant noise of the ward that my brain couldn't fully process what *quiet* sounded like. I was still getting used to the idea that I was free.

It was lunchtime and for the first time in a long while, food sounded good to me. The hotel was popular with divers and had a dive shop attached to it. It was also on the waterfront. Jon and I went to the bar/café area to get some lunch. We were both feeling a little shell-shocked, but in pretty good spirits. We ate lunch by the water and just kind of soaked in what we had been through. We didn't say a whole lot. I ate some kind of chicken dish because I was afraid to try anything too out there. After all, my most recent experiences with food hadn't been so pleasant. Besides, after being on an IV diet for so long, my system couldn't take in too much at one time and I knew Jon liked this dish and would eat what I didn't.

Jon's bartender friend saw us and commented on how good I looked. He was being kind, but all in all, I was alive, upright, and dressed—all big steps forward for this girl! I thanked him for being a friend to Jon during the past few days. Jon and I took a selfie to send to the kids so they could see that I was actually out. We knew they would get it to the rest of the family.

Jon: Whew!! Freed at last. What an ordeal!

Katie: Aghhhhh!!!!!!!!!!!!!! Sunshine!!!!!!!!

Me: Such a HUGE emotional relief.

Jimmy: So glad things r moving in the right directions. What is in the glass? Vodka?

Jon: No, that's water. I had a beer.

Jimmy: Huge relief for us all.

Katie: Enjoy the sunshine and nice, NORMAL bed this evening.

Jimmy: One more day. You guys ready?

Jon: No, we've decided that I should have my appendix out too. See you next week.

I'd been awake and mostly sitting or walking the entire day so far—six or seven hours—and I was exhausted. My muscles felt like they were hanging loosely off my bones. Even though I didn't sleep straight through the night in the ward, I was napping frequently. I needed to take a nap now. Jon helped me get back to the room. It had two double beds in it. He pointed out the one that was the most comfortable and I maneuvered myself into bed to take a nap while he tried to figure out our travel home.

It hit me that I wasn't in the hospital any more with nurses checking on me 24/7 and I was a little worried that if something happened to me we wouldn't catch it until it hit crisis point. I was still breathing very heavy and sometimes I felt like I couldn't catch my breath. Jon was heading out to the front porch of our room to make his travel calls. I asked him to check on me every once in a while, which he quickly agreed to do. As excited as we were to have me out of the hospital, I think it's fair to say that we were both a little worried that something else would happen. I tried to put that out of my mind and concentrated on my breathing mantra, but I couldn't calm my mind. It hit a whole new level of self-awareness. Finally, I was able to absorb the quiet coolness of the room and I dozed on and off for the better part of three hours.

During that whole time, Jon worked hard to make our travel plans. I often think about how lucky I am to be married to him. I startled easily and was in absolutely no condition to handle any kind of controversy. He literally took care of everything without complaining and showed amazing patience with me. He'd even already planned ahead to our travel home when he packed our bags from Citrus Creek! There was one suitcase full of dirty (and now smelly) clothes and one with our rapidly dwindling stash of clean ones.

"Susan was in pretty good spirits Friday afternoon. I called Delta to make arrangements to fly home. Unfortunately (or not, as it turned out), I was not able to get flights back until Monday morning. I wanted two seats together in first class. Susan was still very sore and sitting in anything less than first class would have been too painful for her. As much as we wanted to leave the island, I thought it might not be a bad thing to have a couple extra days of healing before the long day of travel. I also made arrangements to stay at a place close to the airport Sunday night. The drive to the airport was again on slow, winding roads and it would be dark in the wee hours of the morning otherwise. We didn't want to do that. I made arrangements at Coffee River Cottages, the closest lodging of any type I could find in my Internet search for places near the airport. I knew it wouldn't be a typical hotel since each unit was its own cottage and they were set on the bank of a river, but it was all I could find. After reviewing the pictures and write-up, I decided it would suit our needs. After all, we'd only be there overnight."

Jon also checked in with my office. We both knew that everyone there was worried about us and sending prayers and healing energy.

Jon: Susan had a very rough day emotionally yesterday and some allergic reactions to some medication last night. However she has healed well physically and is being released from the hospital today. She's a happy girl. We still need to make travel arrangements so aren't exactly sure what day we will be back. My best guess is Sunday but will let you know for sure. Also, Susan will have her doctor at home review everything once she is back, so next week will likely be filled with medical appointments.

My boss: Goodness, what a journey . . . I hope getting back stateside will lift her spirits and set her on a good path toward healing. Take good care of yourselves. We're not expecting to see you all any time soon, so tell her please not to worry about a thing here. The bases are being covered. Again, if there's any help we can provide with travel arrangements or support when you get home, please do let us know. You all continue in our thoughts and prayers.

When I woke up and the travel plans were made, I knew I needed to walk around. Although I'd been up most of the day, I hadn't maintained my strict hourly walking plan and didn't want my recovery to slip back. I needed to stay on smooth surfaces as much as possible because I still couldn't lift my feet too high and was taking baby steps. I also had some trouble maintaining my balance, so I tried to walk in places where I could grab on to something if needed.

Jon was a good guide and a steady hand. Funny thing . . . Dominica is full of some of the world's most amazing hiking trails, but it's a little light on sidewalks. And with the crazy drivers, I wasn't about to take any chances walking on the road. To resolve the problem, Jon and I found some short loops to do around the hotel property. Then, he suggested that we go to the botanical garden on Saturday, which had some longer walking paths and would be out of the chaos of the city streets , and that sounded nice.

Friday evening, I texted our extended family to let them know I was out of the hospital and doing okay. Jon and the kids had been handling most of the family communication and I had a feeling that they needed to hear from me in addition to the other updates. Support rolled in.

> **Me:** What a journey this has been. I'm out of the hospital and will be traveling Monday to give me a couple of days to recover before a long travel day and to make sure no other issues come up before we cross the island for the airport. I'll share more later, but please know that I really felt your love, prayers, good wishes and concerns. They made a HUGE difference. There are simply no words. Please keep them coming. . . . I have some recovery time ahead and can use all the prayers, prayer chains, prayer groups, good vibes and positive energy, texts and emails. I may not be responding all the time but know that I read them over and over again. I love you all more than I can say.
>
> **Family:** Thinking of you and imagining how glad you are to be out of the hospital and back with Jon in a more peaceful setting. Hope you're able to travel in a wheelchair—it would be a great help, I'm sure.
>
> **Family:** I hope this finds you better than yesterday. I'm not sure what day you will travel back stateside but I wish you well. I have prayed every day for you. Have a safe journey home. I love you. Stay the course! Keep the faith!
>
> **Family:** Just saying that I have always loved you so much Susan and Jon but I don't think we express it enough! This experience has made me reevaluate many important people in my life and communication with family and how important it is!

The kids continued to keep a close eye on both Jon and me.

> **Me:** We are so blessed to have you for our kids. Thank you seems so small, but so powerful. We love you.

Jimmy: What u guys do today?

Jon: Got back to the hotel early afternoon. Then we walked a bit for her exercise, watched the sunset, and had dinner. Mom had a new appreciation for things like flowers and little kids in a park.

Katie: Aw! I'm sure she does.

Jimmy: I think we all probably do on some level.

Jon: Need a wake-up call once in a while to keep things in perspective. Fortunately this one had a happy ending.

Jimmy: Fortunately.

Katie: Next time can we please have less of a severe wake-up call?

Jimmy: Yah!!

Jon: Haha, agreed. There has to be a less anxious way to do this.

Jon sent a final email to my office explaining when we'd be coming home and thanking them for their prayers. We were both so humbled by the love that everyone had shown us throughout our ordeal.

As happy as we were, however, our adventure wasn't quite over yet.

One More Setback

Earlier in the day, I spotted a plastic chair and asked the hotel if I could put it in the shower. I knew I couldn't shower, but there was a sprayer and Jon was going to help me wash my hair. They were happy to help.

I wish I could have seen Jon negotiating with the sprayer, me, the chair, the shampoo, and the towel to keep me dry. It had to have been hilarious. He was so incredibly patient. The shower was a large, zero-entry stone stall that looked like it had recently been remodeled. Jon positioned the chair so I could sit in it and lean over as far as possible (which wasn't that far because it hurt too much). I wasn't being very helpful because I was worried that I'd blow a stitch or accidentally loosen the bandage or get myself soaked. So here I was, not able to see much of anything other than the shower floor tiles and giving directions to Jon about how to wash my hair. I'm lucky he didn't open fire on me with the sprayer!

The water felt heavenly, but the best part was having clean hair. I was also able to use some hypoallergenic facial cleansing wipes I've often used before to wash my body as much as I could. I wasn't squeaky clean, but it was the freshest I'd been in a week!

While this was all going on, I hit a pothole. I broke out into another rash. This one was a little different but still itched like crazy. It seemed to be limited to my arms and legs with nothing on my face or torso. I started to freak out. I cried and showed Jon. My reaction was irrational, but I just couldn't handle anything else. My mind leaped to the worst-case scenario of readmission to the hospital and a delay in getting back home.

I was able to get a hold of myself and we decided to wait and see what was going on with the rash. It seemed more like an allergy than a medical reaction. Jon and I ate a quiet dinner in the open-air restaurant of the hotel. We watched a beautiful sunset and I realized that I hadn't seen one in over a week. It was gorgeous, and the colors seemed more vivid than I remembered. I was really trying to focus on relaxing and I'm glad I did. In addition to the sunset, I was able to enjoy dinner of chicken, French fries, and fresh vegetables. I didn't eat much, but it was the first food that tasted like anything to me in a long time and even better than my lunch earlier in the day. Jon ate what I didn't.

Gradually, night fell and the stars came out. I hadn't seen stars for so long, I was enthralled by the sheer awesomeness of their light and energy. We didn't really say much at dinner. Jon and I were both so overwhelmed by everything we'd been going through. It was starting to hit us, but we both knew we had to keep it together to get home.

Once we were back in the room, I wanted to go to sleep. I was exhausted again. My rash was covering my legs and felt like a million little no-see-um bugs were biting me. I washed down with some wipes, which helped a lot.

The rash was really making me worried, though, so I started texting with Jimmy and Megan, who is a pharmacist. A thought flashed through my mind that I was being unfair to call on Jimmy. He was still in training and while I'm fully confident in his skills, I remembered something about physicians not treating family members because of the pressure of mistakes. However, I no longer had the nurses to rely on. I knew I could call Dr. Theodore, but I was hoping that my anxiety was more about my mind getting the best of me than an actual issue. I also didn't feel in my gut that this was life-threatening. At this point, I'd been on so many drugs I'm sure my body chemistry was really messed up. I decided that I had to trust Jimmy to tell me what the limits of our conversation would be and texted away. I needed his help.

While I waited to hear back from Jimmy, I tried to be rational. I always travel with Zyrtec and thought maybe I could start with that. I was still breathing very heavy and my chest felt weighted down, but I was starting to get used to it and didn't think it was related to this new problem. While I was texting Jimmy and Megan, I was reading through my medical paperwork from the hospital—the same paperwork I had to keep safe so that we could get back to the States.

Megan assured me I could take Zyrtec with the antibiotics I was still taking. Jimmy asked me more about my symptoms and I sent him a picture of my rash. He was careful not to diagnose, but he did point out that with everything I'd been through and my sensitivity to soaps and things that it was likely a contact allergic reaction. I told him I had the doctor's cell phone and Jimmy encouraged me to contact Dr. Theodore if there was any change or if I continued to feel nervous. He reassured me that doctors who give out their cell phone numbers to patients expect to receive a call and are prepared for that at any time of the day or night. He also reminded me that I hadn't survived up to this point by accident.

That last statement kind of got to me. I needed to trust that I was going to be okay. I'd been told when I was in the light that I wasn't going to die, but I was finding it harder and harder to stand up to the recovery I knew was already under way. I was very distraught by anything that could possibly stand between me and going home.

I finished my conversation with Megan and Jimmy, and Jon and I turned out the light. Somehow I found a comfortable spot to sleep in. I asked my spirit team to guide my sleep and my soul.

I was still finding it hard to pray, but I hadn't given up trying to reach out to the universe for support. It was about 10:00 p.m. when I laid my head down, and the next time I woke up, it was 3:30 a.m. and I needed to make a bathroom run. I'd just slept for five hours straight for the first time since the night of my surgery!

My body thanked me, although I realized that it was stiff. I successfully used the bathroom without incident—hooray!—then headed back to bed. I didn't fall asleep for at least an hour. My mind was racing, but I really tried to pray again and have some conversations with my spirit team. I thanked them for getting me to this point and thanked God for having a divine plan for me that is yet to be fulfilled. Oddly, the song "Jesus Loves Me" popped into my head, and I heard the voices of Katie and Jimmy when they used to sing it together at the top of their lungs when they were little kids. I smiled. I relaxed a little. Then I repeated a new mantra breath: *peace enter me* as I inhaled and *negative energy leave me* on the exhalations.

The breathing helped and I fell asleep again. The next time I awoke, it was 7:00 a.m. My body told me that I needed to drink water, which tasted so refreshing to me. I also needed to sit up for a bit. All I kept thinking was, "I'm here. I made it through my first night with a lot of help from my spirit team, my family, Jon, and from myself. One step at a time." I texted the kids after I'd checked in with the doctor to thank them for being my lifeline the previous night. The doctor said that he was in the hospital and to check back in with him if the rash came back. Jimmy told me it was normal to feel a little jumpy and hypochondriacal, all things considered. I felt very fragile, as if I were just a thought or two from a total breakdown.

Jon and I dressed and went to breakfast. The breakfast room was on the second floor. When Jon and I got to the bottom of the stairs, I looked at him and said I wasn't sure I could make it because it was hard to put any kind of pressure on my right leg and my torso couldn't support my weight very well. I grabbed the rail and asked him to spot me from behind. I started to climb. I had to lead with my left foot and kind of drag my right foot along. It was slow going and painful, but I managed.

After breakfast, the owners saw me trying to descend the stairs—another slow process.

"How are you?" the owners asked with looks of great concern on their faces. "We'd be happy to bring breakfast to your patio tomorrow so you don't have to climb the stairs."

"That's so nice of you," I replied. "I'm a little slow, but getting better every day. I'm okay on the stairs. If that changes, I'll be sure to let you know and happily take you up on your offer." We smiled at each other. They were genuinely concerned about me. Their kindness was humbling.

Climbing those stairs was a milestone of sorts for me. I knew intuitively that I needed to keep challenging myself physically (within reason) if I was going to heal. I couldn't do anything about my mental state, which was in survival mode only. I could only connect with my spiritual side through nature and through all those who were praying for me. What seemed more in my control were my physical actions and I was all over them. I concentrated on listening to my body so I didn't overdo it, but I was adamant that I wouldn't take a step backward (no pun intended). I was still walking only a few yards at a time very slowly and by applying reverse pressure on my abdomen, but I was walking. I was also getting used to being in pain and able to handle it better.

I hadn't had any pain meds since my stay in the hospital, even though I had some I could take. Dr. Theodore had told me that I could decide if I needed them and I chose not to take them. Because of the mental state I was in, I didn't trust myself to take anything other than the antibiotics. There's no doubt in my mind the painkillers would have helped with the pain, but I was worried that I'd lose what little ability I felt I had left to think for myself. Besides, I have a high threshold for pain and a poor history of reactions when it comes to taking pain meds. The doctor knew all of this and prescribed pills that would be right for me. I wanted to hold off until I felt I really needed them. I had a feeling that it wasn't going to be easy on my body to travel home. I expected to take them then. Jon agreed with my decision.

We still had two days on the island before we could fly home. It was beautiful weather in a beautiful place, but we really didn't care. We wanted to go home so badly. The rash had subsided from the Zyrtec, but something still didn't feel right. There was just something underneath that nagged at me. The blackness wasn't back, but I was not feeling fully in the light.

Jon was getting worried again.

"She called Dr. Theodore again and explained what was going on. He said he could prescribe something stronger than Zyrtec if necessary. I could tell Susan was an emotional mess. Understandable based on what she had been through for almost a week now. Her upbeat attitude from getting out of the hospital didn't last long. By Saturday she was very quiet and sullen. I was getting concerned again. I asked her if she wanted to go to the botanical garden and walk a little, which she did."

My mental state was becoming confused again. I was worried about the rash. I was worried about the long trip home. I was starting to feel anxious in crowds and around loud noises. I became startled at just about everything. This was a red flag to me because I had never really feared crowds or loud noises. When I would breathe, it felt like the air wasn't completely filling my lungs. I imagined my lungs as sieves with many tiny spaces where air was leaking out instead of filling me up. My voice started to get a little hoarse and I cleared my throat more often.

Jon's suggestion to go to the botanical garden was a good one. I needed to walk around and that place was beautiful. Besides, I was connecting with nature more and something told me that it would be a place of peace.

At the botanical garden, Jon parked the car and helped me to walk across the grass. I was exhausted again so we sat down on a bench and watched some kids play cricket. There were two groups. One was a bunch of little kids who looked like they were about five or six. They seemed to be learning the game for the first time. Their patient coaches made it fun and there was a lot of laughter. It made me smile. Those boys were so excited to be playing cricket. It seemed so simple.

The other group was made up of older boys, maybe age ten or so. They were definitely experienced enough to be competitive with each other. They were fun to watch, too, because they were having so much fun. It was very joy-filling to sit there and watch them. I was reminded of the early sports teams for our own kids and thinking happy thoughts.

The fresh air and sunshine soon tired me out and I laid my head on Jon and dozed.

"While Susan was leaning against me," Jon said, "I envisioned her surrounded in a green healing light. I kept that vision for as long as I could. I don't know if it helped but I figured at this point it couldn't hurt."

When I woke up, I still felt very nervous. I called Dr. Theodore again and told him about the rash, how hard it seemed for me to take a full breath, and the fact that I was having a hard time concentrating. He told me to come back to the hospital so he could meet with me and give me a prescription for something stronger than Zyrtec to help keep the rash at bay. I could tell that he also wanted to see me to check out the other symptoms I described. His tone on the phone didn't suggest that he was concerned, just that he wanted to be very thorough. I was immediately relieved on one front, but still feeling very unsure of myself in general.

Jon, as usual, was with me every step of the way.

"It was a little different this time at the hospital," Jon recalled. "This time Susan could see the full picture of where she had been for the past several days. Dr. Theodore sat us down and prescribed some Benadryl for the rash, which he attributed to something environmental. He also said that he could tell Susan was pretty emotional and wound up. He agreed that she had been through a lot and we should do something like take a drive to relax. Carnival celebrations were about to get under way and he advised us to steer clear of those as they were crowded and tended to get a little rambunctious. It was welcome advice, and while we were there we let him know our travel arrangements and he was able to see her again. Conditions of her release were now met."

Once again, we reported in to the kids that I had added Benadryl to my personal pharmacy and that the doctor didn't seem worried. They were relieved.

We went back to the hotel where I slept and Jon read. I was feeling better about this allergic reaction but had lost my energy and positive attitude. The emotional roller coaster I'd been on for so long had taken a toll on me and I was struggling to stay steady. I felt like I was on the brink of a total meltdown and worried about our travel home. Looking back, I think the trauma and drama of the preceding several days were starting to catch up to me all at once and my mind was trying to process it, without much success.

This "lost" feeling was new for me. I'm usually the person others have counted on. My brain tends to stay sharp during a crisis and I can keep everyone and everything moving. I had always been the consummate multitasker and was very comfortable in that role. My new reality was forced dependency on the mercy and good humor of others. Surrendering this level of control was hard for me and a little scary.

The scariest part was that suddenly the world seemed too big for me. It didn't take much for me to feel sensory overload. I just couldn't tune much out any longer and it felt like I no longer had control over how much to take in. Sensory inputs were coming in fast and furious and my mind and spirit couldn't keep up. I needed to make my world small in order to have any hope of staying connected to it.

Subconsciously, I started to retreat into myself. I got quiet—something rare for me. I kept my eyes shielded from bright light and often closed them. I tried not to listen to anything. I avoided overly seasoned foods. I held Jon's hand, rested my head on his shoulder, or touched his arm frequently as if it were an anchor to my storm. This new Susan was me, but it wasn't the me I was used to. I decided to focus on each moment and then when it passed, the next moment. It sounds simple, but it was actually quite difficult for me to do. I really had to work hard to keep any thoughts from lingering too long. I just didn't have it in me to keep up anymore.

Jon was watching me intently and noticed the change.

"Susan was feeling better about the allergic reaction but still very quiet," he said. "I have never seen her that way before, but I think she was doing everything she could to just eliminate any outside stimulus so she could stay calm. This lasted the rest of the afternoon and through dinner. It was very quiet, but I understood. I was counting the hours until we could leave.

"After we got something to eat in the little bar area and took a short walk, we went back to the room. For some reason I asked where the paperwork from the hospital was. I had put it all into a single envelope. It was all very critical paperwork to potentially get through airport security but also to have for the doctors at home. She had it out the night before when she was telling the kids what medications she was on. She told me that I had it. Then she said she left it on the nightstand between the beds.

"It wasn't there. We tore the room apart trying to find it. It seemed to be gone. The only thing I could think of was that the cleaning person may have thrown it away by mistake. I went to the front desk to ask about the possibility of the trash still being there. I explained what had happened and they got the cleaning person on the phone. He said he had seen an envelope with papers in it along the side of the bed closest to the wall. He had left it there. I went back to the room and there it was, just where he said he saw it. I pulled it out and tossed it on the bed in partial relief but admittedly partial frustration. Susan was already in tears but when I pulled it out she cried more and told me not to trust her with anything important right now. That was the closest I got to feeling panic throughout this entire ordeal."

When Jon said that our medical paperwork was missing, my heart stopped. For a split second, I was confused because I thought he had it. I couldn't think rationally. I started to cry. My brain froze and all I could think about was how we were going to get back to the United States and how I was going to explain everything to my doctors at home. I was utterly defeated. To have come so far and then have this happen just didn't seem fair. Worse yet, I knew it was all my fault. Jon had been so amazing all week. I felt like I'd let him down.

It was a pivotal moment for me. I realized that I couldn't be counted on to be responsible for anything. A-N-Y-T-H-I-N-G. For the girl who was used to being in charge, that was a mighty big, but necessary, blow. In my final act of surrender, once Jon recovered the paperwork, I said, "I'm poison right now. Don't trust me with anything of value. I just can't handle it."

He took charge of everything from that point forward. I just tried to do what I was told.

The Road Home

The next day, Sunday, marked the beginning of two days of travel to get back home. We had our travel plans all set and I was trying hard to rally. I woke up stiff and sore, but thankfully the Benadryl was helping to take some of the edge off my anxiety. I was exhausted and slept a lot, but on the upside, my rash was under control.

We went to breakfast in the usual spot on the second floor. I was still very, very slow on the stairs and needed Jon to spot me, but I wasn't as overwhelmed by them as I had been the day before, which made me feel a sense of accomplishment. I was definitely celebrating the small victories!

In the dining area a large group of more than a dozen divers was eating a big breakfast before heading out to sea. They were very boisterous as they shared adventure stories and plotted their day. If I had been healthy, I'd have talked with them, asked all about their upcoming dive, and wished them well. I'm not a diver, but it fascinates me. Besides, what Jon and I had seen snorkeling early in our vacation was only a glimpse into what they'd be able to see. On this day, it was too much activity for me. Every laugh assaulted my ears as if each person in the group was laughing at the same time at a staccato pace inside my head. My head hurt. My abdomen felt knotted up where I'd had my surgery and each movement felt as if it were pulling on the stitches down deep inside of me.

My skin seemed to absorb the energy of the group and my nerves just below the surface felt like they were shaking. I tried hard to focus on eating. I said my new breathing mantra and waited. No change. To maintain some sense of balance, I repeated in my head the steps I was taking to eat breakfast. Pick up your fork. Scoop up some eggs and potatoes. Put it in your mouth. Chew. Swallow. Get a drink of bottled water. Pick up your fork. . . . I also tried to look out at the beautiful sea as much as possible.

Jon was continuing to watch my every move as today was going to be our last full day in Dominica.

"All we wanted to do was get through the day. Susan was extremely quiet trying to remain calm. She was healing both physically and mentally. The noise of the group was overwhelming to her; that is usually my issue, not hers, so I could relate to some of her feelings. The divers left before we did, so we had some quiet then."

We went back to the room to pack up. As I mentioned earlier, we travel light—one backpack and one medium suitcase each. Jon chose to use his backpack as our joint carry-on and started rearranging the suitcases to fit my pack and its content inside. At this point, we decided to downsize anything that wasn't essential. We knew that the commercial airline back to the States could handle heavier baggage, but we thought the small prop planes getting us off Dominica had stricter regulations. Neither one of us wanted to deal with that headache.

Jon was on a mission to get this right. I was exhausted and mostly sat on the bed answering questions as they came up. I was still very quiet and concentrating on maintaining some level of self-awareness. We really hadn't bought anything big to take back, but because we were consolidating our belongings by one backpack, our luggage was a lot more crowded than when we'd arrived. We decided to give our snorkel gear to the man who'd cleaned our room and saved our medical paperwork. It was taking up some much-needed real estate. Jon went to track down the young man, who seemed genuinely surprised and appreciative of our gesture. We were just glad he could use it.

After all that sensory overload, I needed a nap. I slept and Jon read out on the porch. We had agreed that we would eat lunch at the hotel and then begin the one-hour trek across the island to our hotel near the airport. We were keeping things simple.

From Jon:

"After lunch we settled the bill and said good-bye to all of the people at Castle Comfort who had been so kind to us during our stay there. They truly were wonderful hosts and made us feel very much at home. I felt like they were our friends."

Checking out of the hotel was both easy and hard for me. On the one hand, it was a haven of sorts for Jon and for me. It was also a known entity. Neither one of us had any idea of what we'd be walking into in our next place by the airport. On the other hand, I was almost giddy at the thought that we were starting our journey home. It didn't seem real and I was afraid to believe that we actually had a shot at getting off the island. Too much had happened.

I wasn't looking forward to this drive. First, every single pothole, start, stop, and turn made my core hurt. There's no way to soften that. It felt like I was getting punched in the gut over and over and over again. The reverse pressure helped with some of the intensity of the spikes of pain, but it still hurt. A lot. Second, the roads made me nervous when I was in good health. Facing them at this time was almost too much to think about. Finally, I was still having difficulty sitting up for long periods of time. Sitting more or less upright for an hour seemed like a long stretch and I wasn't sure how I'd hold up.

I still held off on taking the pain meds Dr. Theodore prescribed. Looking back on it, I think I underestimated my need to take them. That was a big mistake. According to the doctor, I was healing just fine, but I think I might have slept better and held up better under all of the pressure. Most important? It just wouldn't have hurt as much.

We stopped for some groceries and got gas in the car before heading across the island. Neither one of us was too crazy about cooking that night, but we also didn't want to take a chance that there wouldn't be a restaurant nearby. Besides, I wasn't sure what kind of shape I'd be in after such a long ride. I eased myself into the car again, put my seat back as far as it would go so I could sit at about a forty-five-degree angle, strapped myself in, and gently pushed on my middle. I focused on my breathing mantra and kept telling myself that I was getting closer and closer to home. I didn't say much and eventually drifted in and out of sleep.

Jon had become an expert road warrior by this time. He was taking extra care to make the drive as easy on me as possible.

"Earlier in the week when riding in the car on these roads Susan was very stressed. These types of roads are not her thing. Her hands are usually clenched tightly together to the point of getting cramped. This time she seemed much more relaxed. I don't know if it was because she was trying hard to stay calm or if I was driving much slower so as not to make her incision move and hurt her. Regardless of the reason, she seemed to handle the drive much better."

It took a little over an hour to get to the cottage. We found the turnoff to the cottage and started up the road. Notice that I said *up the road*. The cottage was located on the property of a working banana plantation. The road was little more than a path that had been cut out of the bush and was wide enough for a small truck. It was mostly filled with rocks and potholes. There were banana trees growing all along the road. And, the trek was uphill. We prayed that our little car would make it.

Jon looked at me with sympathy. We both knew that we had to keep going, but he also knew that in doing so he was going to contribute to my pain. I took a deep breath, applied more pressure, and looked out the window. I was focused on not gasping or crying out (which I had done already on the trip across the island—even though I was trying not to) because I didn't want to add to Jon's self-imposed burden. He was doing such a great job of getting us where we needed to be while at the same time managing me.

When we got to the cottage, we learned that it was a little guest house next to the main residence of an older couple. The wife was British and her husband was from Australia. Their place was an eco-residence, which meant they were largely self-sustaining when it came to water, power, and food. When I got out of the car, their dog came rushing up. I couldn't handle the thought that it might jump up on me. I stuck close to the car while Jon intercepted the dog.

The couple came out to talk with us and realized that something was wrong with me.

"Are you okay?" they asked with great concern showing on their faces. "Do you need anything?"

I didn't answer immediately. Jon came to my rescue.

"She's recovering from surgery for a ruptured appendix," he said. "She's going to be fine, but she just got out of the hospital a few days ago."

"You were in the hospital in Roseau?" They looked genuinely shocked that I was alive, but not because of the appendix. "You were lucky. We've never heard of anyone saying they'd received good care there. We haven't had to deal with anything life-threatening so we haven't been there, but when we need procedures, we go to Canada."

Jon and I listened politely but dismissed their comments. I felt I had to stand up for the hospital and my medical team on the spot. "That wasn't my experience at all," I said. "They saved my life. I received excellent care from every single person I met."

The couple graciously accepted what I said and offered again to help in any way they could. They were very kind to us and even checked in on me a few times just to make sure I was settling in all right.

We pulled up to our cottage. It was another true Caribbean-style open-air building with no air conditioning. We'd assumed that there would be air conditioning, but at this point anything that didn't go according to plan was no longer surprising to us. This had been anything but a typical vacation.

While I agreed that we needed to drive across the island the day before our flight rather than trying to negotiate the roads in the dark on a set schedule, my spirits sank as I walked in. The cottage was nicely decorated and spotless. What didn't work so well for me was that the bathroom was on the first floor while the bedrooms were on the second floor, located up ladder-like steps to an open-air loft. Big, glassless, unscreened windows flanked either side of the loft, which meant we'd essentially be camping indoors. The first floor had a small loveseat and a chair. The main living space, like most Caribbean homes, was located outside. Where Castle Comfort was close to a typical American-style hotel, Coffee Cottages was exactly what it promoted, Caribbean-style cottages in a serene setting on the banks of a river. If I wanted to sleep in a bed, I had to become an expert ladder climber in my unstable condition. Suddenly those stairs at the hotel in Roseau didn't look so intimidating!

I started to panic again at the thought of having to navigate down the steps in the dark to go to the bathroom. My body was craving water and I was taking in as much as I could. I was also using the bathroom a lot. As I thought about this next challenge, my chest got heavier. My lungs felt like they were being squeezed. My brain started back into its bulletlike rhythm. Ugh.

Jon felt the same way I did. He took one look at the stairs and I could see real concern on his face. I mustered myself quickly because I didn't want him to worry all night. I knew I'd be up a lot, but he needed to get some sleep in order to get us home the next day. I just wasn't up to managing any travel of that magnitude myself. I showed him how I thought I could climb up and down the stairs. Up was slow but steady, like what I'd done in our previous hotel. To get down, however, I had to go backward. I literally had to back down while holding on to the railing. It was slow going, but I was able to do it. I'm still not sure that Jon was fully confident in my abilities, but his face relaxed. A little.

I needed to walk a bit since I'd been sitting so long in the car. Sitting was still the worst position for me to be in because my middle simply couldn't support my body for very long and it felt like my stitches were under strain. I had no strength and I hurt a lot. The property was a gorgeous setting and there was a little river near the cottage. If I'd been healthy, I would have wanted to wade in it or follow it to see where it ended up. Some rain was coming in, so our walk was cut short. The walkway was slightly uneven, so I was holding on to Jon to stay steady.

Suddenly, Jon pointed to the sky. He'd been keeping an eye on the dark clouds approaching. When I looked up, however, it wasn't dark clouds that I saw. It was a rainbow in all its colorful glory. It had a perfect arch to it and was one of the most beautiful sights I'd ever seen. I immediately started crying. It felt like a sign from the universe that everything was going to be okay. It felt like our journey home was being blessed and that felt good.

Jon fixed dinner while I rested on the lanai. I didn't eat much, but it was enough. Then, Jon packed up as many of our things as he could. He showered and I washed up with my facial wipes and we went to bed. I'm not sure that either one of us expected to get much sleep. We were in separate single beds, which was fine with me. It was too hot and humid to sleep together. Besides, I didn't want anything to bump into my stitches.

As I was lying in bed, the jungle noises all around us got louder and louder to me. While these had been soothing when we started our vacation in this island paradise, they no longer represented comfort to me. I could feel myself heading back into high-anxiety mode. All I could think about was the open, screenless windows. I hate bats and I had these visions in my head of bats flying in and out of the cottage. I even had a flash of a snake slithering in from a nearby tree.

I felt like I could barely breathe, I was so scared. Jon seemed to be sleeping fine over on his side of the room. I focused on my peaceful breathing mantra. I even tried to visualize the letters of the words I was saying in my head in an attempt to rid my brain of the scary images. Eventually, my mind went blank and the imagery stopped. I clutched a small flashlight Jon had given me to use when I was going up and down the stairs because the house was pitch black. Thankfully, the blackness I'd experienced before was nowhere to be seen. It was my imagination getting the best of me. That I could deal with.

To keep out the night critters, we'd been instructed to close all doors and shutter the windows on the first floor. For airflow, we were to keep the shutters on the second-story windows open. The care and handling of this organic environment was just not something I was up for. I wanted walls that connected to ceilings. I wanted screens on windows. I wanted to be able to drink water from the tap. I wanted to be able to shower without worrying about getting a rash. I just wanted to go home.

Unbeknownst to me at the time, Jon was struggling with his own uncertainties that night.

"It rained pretty hard, the wind was blowing, and it was humid. Susan said she saw things flying through the loft that night. I didn't see anything, but I heard some bugs on the wall next to my bed. Sleep was hard to come by. I had thoughts of getting back down that road in the morning. What if the car didn't make it after all of this? What if we got a flat tire? What if we missed the plane? Lots of travel anxiety. I managed to get a little sleep, but Susan said she didn't sleep much at all. It didn't really matter at that point. We were just waiting for the alarm to go off so we could get up and leave. We had an eight o'clock flight the next morning. The airport was only a mile away but we had to plan on about fifteen minutes to get there because of the road, and our hosts recommended arriving ninety minutes early.

"The 5:00 a.m. alarm rang. We were both out of bed quickly. I'm usually good for lying there a bit before getting up, but not this time. We were both up and in full travel mode instantly. Susan was moving slowly because of her condition, so there wasn't much she could help with. I fixed something for us to eat, cleaned up the dishes and kitchen, packed everything up, made sure all paperwork was ready, packed the car, and so on. We were out of there by about six o'clock."

I was slower than usual that morning. I was tired from lack of sleep, tired from the recovery process, and generally feeling poorly. It had been only one week since my surgery and I was completely spent from the whole ordeal. My skin and muscles felt like they were hanging from my bones. My brain was also in a state of turmoil again. I kept myself very quiet and tried to shore up as much as possible for the travel day. We would literally be traveling for about eighteen hours across two islands, two countries, and four airports and on three planes, two cars, and whatever other modes of transportation we needed to get through the airports. I knew I'd have to be sitting up for most of the day and I wasn't looking forward to it at all. My core was not strong enough to support me for that much sitting without a lot of pain. My salvation was knowing that we were headed home.

I folded myself back into the car and got as comfortable as I could be knowing the kind of road conditions we were facing. We could see the airport from the hillside where the cottage was located, but we had to drive out of the jungle to get to it.

Daylight was just starting, so the bumpy road wasn't completely dark. Jon went as slowly as he could and the drive out did seem to go faster than the drive in, but that road was bad! At one point a truck filled with plantation workers and their machetes came roaring past us and coasted into the jungle. I couldn't get off this island fast enough.

It was a lot harder to get out of Dominica than it had been to get in. We had to pass through a couple of security gates and pay an exit tax. Our flights were Dominica–San Juan (where we would go through US Customs)–Atlanta–Detroit then a one-and-a-half-hour drive home to Ohio. At that point I wanted to (a) enter the United States no matter where it was and (b) get to Atlanta. Jon's sister and my best friend live there, so if we encountered any problems whatsoever, I knew that all we had to do was contact them. They'd take care of both of us.

We said good-bye to our car and left it in the parking lot for Hervé. That little car had stood up to some intense use over the past two weeks. Leaving it was unnerving as we were now at the mercy of someone else for transportation until we got to Detroit. After all the uncertainties of the past seven days, that didn't exactly sit well with me.

I was walking under my own power; no wheelchairs were available. Jon was pulling our two suitcases and wearing his backpack. He was also handling all paperwork and exit taxes. I simply followed along, as I didn't trust myself to do anything other than walk from one point to another and take care of my own needs. It was time to rally.

Our flight would be on a small propeller plane that seated about forty passengers. There weren't many people waiting, but it took nearly an hour to get through the check-in line because multiple flights were leaving in quick succession. There were no chairs, so I left the line after about ten minutes and leaned against the front wall of the ticketing area. I was worried that someone would think I was sick and not let me board the plane, so I tried as much as possible not to look too bad. There was only so much I could do, though. I was kind of bent over and had my hand protectively over my lower abdomen where my stitches were still healing under the massive bandage that had been put on in the hospital. Jon stayed in line with our bags and paperwork. The people at the counter were very slow and it seemed that everyone ahead of him had some special issue that needed to be addressed.

Eventually we made it through all the necessary security gates, tax payments, and other hurdles and were ready to board the plane. We had to wait a few minutes before boarding began, and we ran into the young man Jon had met at Castle Comfort Lodge in Roseau. He was continuing his pre–Peace Corps travels and greeted Jon warmly. He also asked how I was doing. I could see the genuine affection he had for Jon and concern for me. I felt good knowing that Jon had been surrounded by such good people when he most needed a substitute family.

Soon, it was time to go. An airline official lined us up on the tarmac and took us out to the freestanding steps that had been put in place for us to board the plane. The steps were steep (or seemed that way to me), but after my experience at our last cottage, I knew I could make it.

We were toward the end of the line, since we were moving slower than the rest of the people. One woman was pushing an elderly gentleman in a wheelchair behind us. She wasn't paying attention and hit me in the back of the leg with the wheelchair, which startled and upset me. I was exhausted from recovery and lack of sleep, my mind was on high alert, and I could barely stand on my own. I quietly gasped and Jon turned around ready to pounce on the lady behind me. I put my hand on his arm as a signal that I was okay, and we headed toward the steps to board.

The plane was tiny and we couldn't stand up all the way in it. With forty passengers trying to fit in such a small space, it was chaotic. At one point, a young woman with a backpack over her shoulder swung around and hit me square in the stomach with her bag as she searched for her seat. I immediately gasped and hunched over, clutching the seats next to me. I took some quick deep breaths to calm myself down and applied reverse pressure. I also checked to make sure Jon hadn't seen it. I figured he'd go off on this woman and I didn't want to be escorted off the plane, further extending our stay on the island. We found our seats and, in a reversal of our usual seating on a plane, I sat by the window and Jon on the aisle. I needed to rest my head on the window and he wanted to protect me from any unnecessary jostling.

Jon and I looked at each other as the plane taxied down the runway to take off. The G-force of takeoff was painful, but I was able to breathe through it as I had virtually no strength to withstand it physically. The seats were small with very little legroom. I couldn't sit with my legs properly aligned because there wasn't enough distance between my seat and the seat in front of me, even with knees bent. I kind of folded myself up, grabbed my abdomen, and alternated leaning my head against the window and against Jon. When we took off, I cried tears of exhaustion, relief, and joy that we'd made it that far. We were on our way home.

———

Jon was so incredibly protective of me on the trip home and I felt insulated as much as possible from the usual frenzy associated with travel.

I slept on and off for the whole ninety-minute flight to Puerto Rico. It was loud and bumpy. My abdomen felt like it was being pushed and pulled any number of ways. When it was time to land, I braced myself for the pain. As the plane touched down in San Juan, I felt each wheel hit the runway. Bump. Bump. Bump. I recovered as best I could as we taxied to the airport, then cried again. We were back in the United States! It was still an island, but we were getting closer to home. I felt so grateful to have made it this far.

The plane parked on the tarmac and we exited last to avoid the craziness. I was moving slowly and looking for the wheelchair that we had requested. It was nowhere in sight. I sighed, grabbed Jon's arm, and we started to follow the walkway toward the building and Customs. There was no way I could walk on my own at this point. Every step felt like it was pulling at the muscles all along my incision sites. I was back to my shuffling walk one small step at a time from my early hospital days. The distance along the tarmac to the main building was several hundred yards.

Airline personnel saw that I was having trouble walking and brought a wheelchair to come out and get me. I eased myself into the chair and surrendered my mobility to a very nice young man who said he'd stay with us until we got through Customs and to Delta Airlines.

When we pulled up to Customs, Jon gave me my passport and medical paperwork in case I needed it. Since I was in a wheelchair, we were able to go through a special line and didn't have to wait, and we both approached the agent at the same time. I had a baseball hat on, my glasses on, and my hair up in a ponytail. I looked very little like the photo on my passport.

The Customs agent looked back and forth between my passport and me.

"Where have you been?" he asked both Jon and me at the same time. I didn't trust myself to do a lot of talking and remained quiet. Jon told him about our vacation.

"Can you please take off your hat and glasses?" the agent said to me. I immediately complied and the agent again looked back and forth between me and my passport. I was a little nervous at this point, but just sat still and smiled as much as I could.

"Welcome back to the United States," the agent said as he stamped our passports and handed them back to us. He never once asked about my health or to see any medical paperwork.

I didn't realize what a huge relief it would be to get through

Customs. I was more worried than I'd realized until we literally walked through to the *United States*. As we crossed over, I started to cry again. I was so incredibly relieved to be *home*. At this point, my brain was able to focus a little bit. The man helping us wheeled me to the Delta counter; Jon handed me our travel information and asked me if I thought I could handle getting us checked in. I was skeptical but told him I'd take care of it. The Delta ticket agent called for one of Delta's wheelchairs and I was transferred over to the care of Delta. Our original helper took Jon over to another inspection area for our bags to go under an agricultural review. Once that was done, Delta escorted us to our gate.

Jon was relieved as well.

"Once we made it through US Customs it was another big relief. Susan started to cry again. We had about four hours in San Juan, so we decided to go to an airport restaurant for something to eat."

Sitting in the restaurant felt strangely normal. My pain was under control and I felt more like myself than I had in over a week. I ate more food than I had in a week, too, and it actually tasted good. I was still drinking bottled water. No way was I taking any chances on anything that wasn't sealed until I was back on the mainland.

As we sat at the table, both Jon and I were overcome by everything that had happened to us. We looked at each other and teared up. I was on the verge of losing it because I allowed myself to really think about things. I realized how much I owed my survival to Jon. I just love this man so much. While the medical team took care of my physical ailments, Jon had stood guard over my mind and spirit—a much harder job, in my opinion. I started to tell Jon that he had saved my life as much as the doctors had. In that moment, my love for Jon deepened more than I thought possible.

While we've always felt a strong and unexplainable connection—even when we've disagreed—my love bubbled up within me in a new way. It started as a warm glow from the depths of my soul and spread to every fiber of my being. My brain fog lifted another notch and gave me a moment of clarity. I realized that my spirit, which had felt intangible during all of this, had been held in a sacred space by Jon on my behalf. He was both nurturing and guarding my spirit at the same time. It was as if he'd seen through all the pain, suffering, uncertainty, and angst of the past week and raised a shield to protect me when I couldn't protect myself or connect with the very essence of my being. I was overcome but trying to hold it together in the very public restaurant. We still had a long way to go to get home.

The drama of our experience was catching up with Jon, too.

"Things started to hit me while we were sitting there. We were both trying to hold things together for the trip home. Susan had had a few emotional releases since the surgery, but I really hadn't other than Friday morning after she told me she was being released from the hospital. I had a beer in front of me at the restaurant and we had just finished eating. I was sitting there holding a napkin over my mouth with tears in my eyes thinking about what we had just been through. I was trying hard not to break down. Susan started to thank me for everything she said I had done for her, and that I had saved her life as much as the doctors had. I could feel myself ready to lose my composure, so I told her, 'Not yet.' I needed to hold things together until we got home. She understood."

We returned to our gate area to wait for our flight. I alternated walking with lying in some very uncomfortable plastic airport chairs during the rest of our layover in San Juan. I'd now been awake for more time at once than I had for the better part of one week and I was exhausted. I also had been upright or seated rather than lying down and my body was starting to rebel. I hurt but tried not to think about it too much. My mind started playing some tricks on me, too, and became clouded again. The brief reprieve I'd had during lunch was gone. I couldn't focus long enough to read anything. The words on the page would become a jumbled mess. All I could really do was look aimlessly out the window or at the people in the airport.

Finally, they called our flight. Luckily, we were able to board the plane early to take more time to settle in. Our seats were in the front row with plenty of extra room. I could barely stay awake, but I didn't want to look sick and be kicked off the plane. I was on a mission to get back on the mainland and wanted nothing to stop me. I eased myself into my seat as the flight attendant came over to take our drink orders. I was able to snag a pillow, put it against my side, and strap it in with a loose seatbelt so that I had a temporary pressure bandage. It made a big difference. I knew that there was going to be a meal, so I tried to stay awake long enough to eat something. I also drank as much bottled water as I could manage. I was having trouble staying hydrated and felt very dried out.

I continued to struggle focusing my mind. The motion on the television screen in front of me was making me dizzy. To cope, I looked out the window or sat with my eyes closed to reduce as much sensory input as possible. Once I'd eaten, I settled in for a nap and slept for most of the next five hours. I awoke only to use the restroom, drink more water, and change positions. It was just about the best sleep I'd had in over a week. Jon kept watch from his aisle seat right next to me.

When we landed in Atlanta, I woke up and was once again overcome with emotion. Atlanta had been my goal for so long. Our plane landed and tears immediately ran down my cheeks. It felt so good to be so much closer to home.

We'd been worried about the distance between gates in Atlanta because we had less than one hour to change planes, but the universe smiled on us. Our plane to Detroit was boarding right across the corridor from our arrival gate.

At this point, the fog in my brain was on the rise. I started seeing psychedelic images in rapid succession again, which made me feel off balance, even though I was able to walk in a straight line. I needed quiet and to rest my body without it getting jostled. Jon guided me to the next plane and we boarded our last flight. We were in the home stretch of this long journey.

———

The family had been sending us their good wishes for safe travels via text and email. Some we received before we left Dominica. Some we couldn't access until we got to San Juan and others in Atlanta. Their love and support were very real and we felt every bit of it surrounding us in bright light and positive energy as we traveled home. Somehow, knowing that so many were making the journey with us—at least in prayer or thought—was a great comfort.

Unbeknownst to us, Katie, Jimmy, and Megan had worked out how to best help on the home front. Mike was unable to come due to his work and school schedule.

Katie: I just got my work schedule cleared to make sure I'm at your house when you get home Monday. Mema and I are shopping earlier that day to make sure your fridge is stocked with some detailed foods from Jimmy to help with sensitivity to a healing stomach! I know you'll go to bed right away so I will make sure your sheets are clean and the house is at your ideal frigid temperature.

Me: That's so nice! One thing you can take off the list ... changed our bed the day we left. It's fresh and clean (along with other beds). Thank you both so much.

Jimmy: Megan and I are locked into our schedules, unfortunately. Next week is my last week in psych and I have exams as well. We will be there next weekend, though, to visit and hang out

Katie: Ok. Cool, I don't know how to use your washer anyway ;) How am I not going to squeeze you when I hug you!? I'll squeeze Dad extra hard I guess. Jimmy, Megan, and I are there as YOUR CHILDREN, not guests. We are there to help you guys. We will do whatever you want or need, and keep you company and watch movies with you.

Jon: Lol. Just stick your butt out so you don't squeeze her belly and only her shoulders.

Mema: Wow, what a great support team for your parents!!

The flight to Detroit was easy and uneventful. We landed in Detroit and shed a few more tears. I felt like a weight had been lifted off me and the post-trauma exhaustion was starting to set in. I happily got into a wheelchair so we could get our baggage and head to the parking lot. The calendar had flipped to February, and I'd forgotten to put a winter coat in the car. Jon's was there. He quickly put his hat on and wrapped me in his coat. It felt like a warm blanket and was just what I needed. I reclined my seat, buckled my seat belt, and closed my eyes. When Jon got in the car, he looked at me and said, "Let's go home." I cried again.

We texted the family to let them know we were in Detroit.

Mema: Welcome home. Sure u r glad 2 b home. Let me know if I can help out. Do not want to bug u.

Jon: Thanks, Meem. You have no idea what a relief it is to be home. Can't believe we are actually here. Makes all the difference in the world.

Jon: Funny how being in a beautiful warm place just really didn't matter this past week. We just want to be home!!!

Katie: ALMOST HOME!!!!

Jimmy: Detroit. Beautiful this time of year. One more leg of the trip. Can someone text me when you're all home please?

I dozed all the way to our house but saw the sign at the Ohio state line. It's funny . . . I have crossed that line many, many times going to and from the airport. I even worked in Michigan for five years and crossed it twice a day. That said, I felt like I was crossing the state line for the first time ever. It felt like I'd received a gift. I was so grateful to be able to be going home.

When we pulled into our long driveway, I breathed a huge sigh of relief. I could see Jon relax, too. Katie was at the house to greet us. It was late and we'd been up for about eighteen hours and were spent. She immediately hugged both of us.

I experienced that hug in slow motion similar to a movie set where two long-lost family members suddenly find each other for the first time and come together. I'd walked into the house with Jon then looked up and saw Katie's beautiful, smiling face. I could see the worry on it and her joy at seeing both of us alive and standing in front of her. That joy was close to the joy I'd felt when I was bathed in light during my out-of-body experience. It was so amazing to see that in person instead of through the haze of illness.

I could sense that she was hesitant to reach out to me even as she was doing just that. We were both teary-eyed. I tried to grab her first to silently reassure her that I wouldn't break. As our bodies came together, I just let go and sank into her embrace, which was filled with the raw emotions of pure, unconditional love and relief for both of us. We clung to each other and cried. I knew I didn't have to keep it together any longer. We'd had support all along the way from many seen and unseen angels, but knowing that one of the people we're closest to was there to take on some of our burdens was one of the most comforting feelings I've ever had. We. Were. Home.

Keeping It Simple

As I mentioned, circumstances prevented Jimmy and Megan from coming in from Cincinnati until the following weekend. While I know that was very hard for him, it was actually the best thing for me to have the staggered visits.

Once I got home, everything from the past week hit me all at once. I had to accept a lot of help from family and friends. To do that, I reminded myself of the one-year period in which Jon and I had both lost our fathers. So many people wanted to help our families during that time it was truly humbling. I don't think we cooked for a month after each man died! More important, I learned to say yes to everyone who wanted to show their support in some way. From food to rides to calls and notes of support to the extended family to prayers, hugs, and visits—all of it was critical to our family's ability to move forward during the worst of times. Looking back on it, I think that was a training exercise of sorts for me for my own drama. Once again, the universe was conspiring to take care of me even before I knew I needed it.

That first night home felt like heaven. I was in my own bed. I had my own bathroom. I could drink water from the tap. These seemed like such gifts. I had a renewed appreciation for the simplicity of it all. Yet, my brain was still racing. It switched on and off between nervousness and confusion. I was having trouble thinking in full sentences and my thoughts were very scattered.

Jimmy checked in on me first thing the morning after we got home.

Me: Good first night home although woke up a few times and forgot where I was. Thought I was still in Dominica.

Jimmy: Did u wake up in a panic? Or just confused.

Me: Confused at first then nervous then fought through it. Feel ok though, just a bit nervy. Never panic.

Jimmy: Understandable. Very traumatic experience just happened to u.

Me: I know. It's going to take some time. Slow and steady one step forward at a time.

Jimmy: It'll get better. How long are u off work?

Me: TBD but as long as I need. No issues whatsoever there.

Katie was anxious to help and fixed me a wonderful breakfast of eggs, oranges, and yogurt. She even arranged the orange slices decoratively on the yogurt! I knew I needed to walk and she and Jon agreed to accompany me up and down the driveway. Since it's nearly a quarter-mile long through the woods, I knew I could walk in peace and quiet without worrying about traffic or other people. I decided I needed to walk that path once a day.

That first walk was hard. I could barely make it. I felt so stiff and sore. In addition to the surgery site, the gnawing pain in my right hip from the bursitis hurt a lot every time I walked. I held on to Jon's arm to steady me as I was afraid of falling on the uneven ground. The weather was unseasonably warm for February, but it was still colder than the tropical climate I'd just come from.

In spite of the discomfort, that first walk also felt like a gift. As we made our way along the driveway, I noticed things in our woods that I'd taken for granted. The trees were bare but stood proud and tall, quietly guarding the ground below. The birds were singing a little louder than I remembered for the winter. It sounded like a song just for me and made me smile. The wind was cool, but it caressed my skin and made me feel very much alive.

The half-mile round-trip took about forty-five minutes. When I got back to the house, I was exhausted and had to take a nap. Katie wanted to help with something and I asked her to clean out the fridge. Since we'd been gone a week longer than planned, there was some spoiled food in there and the whole thing seemed like it was full of germs, which freaked me out a little bit. I don't think she really liked that job, but she did it without complaining. It was sparkling when she was done and much cleaner than it would have been if I'd done it on my best day.

Jon's mother had brought over some of her delicious homemade chicken soup, which really hit the spot for us. Katie jumped in to make some other foods from scratch, which were delicious and from an approved food list that Jimmy and she had designed to support good gut health and my recovery. She made a lot so that we'd have plenty to eat after she had to go back to Chicago.

If all that wasn't enough, one of the best things she did for me was to help me wash my hair. I was so tired of being slimy. I still had my stitches and wasn't allowed to take a bath. I hadn't yet been to my doctor in the United States and was still strictly following the instructions from my surgeon in Dominica. Clean hair was the one thing I thought I could manage. Katie gathered all the necessary supplies and brought them to the kitchen sink. We'd decided it would be easiest for her to help me there. I was able to lean over the sink and balance myself by holding onto the counter. Katie gently put a towel around my shoulders, wetted my hair, lathered, and rinsed. When she was done, I sat down with my head wrapped up in a towel. I was able to dry my own hair while Katie kept a watchful eye on me. The whole experience was so refreshing and helped me feel a little closer to normal. To this day it stands out as one of the kindest things anyone has ever done for me.

My days had fallen into a pattern of eating a little, drinking a lot of water and herbal tea, walking, and sleeping. I couldn't focus enough to do much reading, and watching television wasn't very appealing. I also needed a lot of quiet. I think I was experiencing some type of PTSD because the magnitude of what had happened to Jon and to me was at the forefront of my mind.

My first instinct was to squelch the feelings. Then, in a moment of true inspiration, I realized I needed to just go with it to start to restore my mind-body-spirit balance. I was so discombobulated that I felt adrift mentally. I had a hard time finishing thoughts and sentences. Often, I'd be speaking and stop midsentence, not able to find the word to go on. Jon was good at picking up the conversation at that point. Then, I would recover and continue. I was also very emotional and often felt on the verge of tears. I was so grateful to be alive and at home. Plus, I very much wanted to feel better. It never occurred to me that I wouldn't recover; I just had to take it one day at a time.

At dinner our first day back, Katie, Jon, and I bowed our heads in prayer just like we always do before a meal.

"Bless, O Lord, this food to our use and us to thy service," I began. Suddenly, I was overtaken by the power of my own spirit and the universe.

"I ask your particular blessings on the many people who lovingly cared for Jon and for me while we were in Dominica," I continued. "I also ask your blessings on our family and friends at home who have worried about us, prayed for us, and offered to help. We are grateful beyond words for their love and support." I paused as tears welled up and my voice cracked. "Thank you for keeping me alive so that I can be here now, in this moment, to receive your love through others. You have surrounded us with grace in more ways than we'll ever be able to count . . ."

At that point, I couldn't continue. I started to cry. Jon cried. Katie cried. They both came over to hug me and I felt so loved in the comfort of their embrace. It was raw and real.

Katie was able to stay only two nights. I decided I needed to do something kind of silly to get out of my own head and to try to bring some focus in. Katie, Jon, and I watched *The Secret Lives of Pets*, an animated comedy on Pay-Per-View. It was just what I needed. I laughed, really laughed, while Katie and I shared a blanket on the couch.

Offers to come and visit or help were pouring in. Unfortunately, I couldn't always accept them. I needed quiet and couldn't handle being around anyone except Jon and the kids. Jon's mom brought us food and checked in on Jon regularly, but I couldn't visit with her either. My office was feeding us for a few days with Jon as the go-between. The food was delicious and beautifully presented. We could taste the love, care, and concern that went into making it.

Recently, at work, I'd come across the phrase "Food is medicine, food is love" at a conference for chefs and foodservice professionals. At the time, I thought it was a good tagline for the conference; but after our experience in Dominica, this phrase took on new meaning. Nourishment is essential for living; but the act of feeding people is essential for a good life. As we ate the food prepared for us, I'd think about the people who'd put it together. I could picture their faces. Their smiles. Their hands making it or deciding what to purchase. It was as if each one was giving me a hug. I vowed not to take these simple acts of kindness and generosity for granted ever again.

For the first two weeks, I needed to be in quiet—almost silence—so that I could start to bring myself back into some state of normalcy. My brain was having a hard time relaxing. Jimmy told me that my fight-or-flight reflex had been on such a high state of alert for so long that I needed to give myself time to catch back up with myself.

My best friend sent me a mix of healing and energy stones. I added them to a gift that we share back and forth with each other to show our support and arranged it in a prominent place in the house for maximum impact. I could tell that the stones were working almost immediately as a renewed sense of calm came over the house. I also felt her love and concern. We've been through a lot over our thirty-five-plus-year friendship. I knew that she wanted with every fiber of her being to come to our house to help take care of me and to support Jon. One of the greatest gifts she's ever given me, however, was the gift of staying in Atlanta and being a support system from afar. She completely understood that I needed quiet and rest and to keep my world incredibly small in order to heal. These stones remain in my home office and continue to send me positive energy and love.

Our friends and family circles were almost as excited and relieved as we were that I was home. They were anxious to see me, but with Jon standing guard, completely understood that I needed space and time. I told them that this had been one of the hardest experiences of my life and reassured them I was getting better each day. Their positive energy and prayers were working. They also kept up of a steady stream of texts.

After Katie left, I hit my first walking milestone. I was nervous about falling and still feeling very unsteady, but I was able to walk without holding on to Jon. He accompanied me solely as a spotter. I felt like I'd won a race. Walking under my own power was very energizing to my spirit and empowered me to keep setting new goals for my recovery.

Jimmy and Megan arrived at the end of our first week home. Like Katie, Jimmy's first hug was all-encompassing. His eyes were full of tears and relief at seeing me for the first time. This hug came at me in slow motion, too. It was as if we each needed that physical connection to reassure ourselves that I was alive. We both let out sighs of gratitude. In that moment, as with his sister, I saw him as both my son and as a caring adult. Megan gave me a big hug as well and I could tell that she'd been through a lot, too, supporting Jimmy. Her face showed so much loving concern for him and relief that he was finally seeing me again after such a scare. It was very emotional for all of us. Both Megan and Jimmy were surrounded by a white glow, like the one I saw with Katie. Again, I didn't question it. I simply took it all in and was so thankful to be able to be present in the moment with them.

Jimmy took me through his usual list of clinical questions. It was very comforting, as my doctor's appointment wasn't for another few days. Once Jimmy was assured that I was progressing, he and Megan settled in for a visit. They walked with me up and down the driveway. They also cooked a delicious dinner of salmon, potatoes, and Brussel sprouts. The whole time I could feel him watching me intently, as if he were making sure that I was still here in the flesh and that I really was recovering. Jimmy and Megan were in the middle of planning their wedding and it was nice to talk about something joy-filled. We watched a stupid movie, and it all seemed so normal. Their visit was just what I needed.

Checking In
with the Doctor

The first week I was home, I called my primary doctor. I go to a family practice and since I usually enjoy good health, I hadn't been there in a while. I've been going to this practice for more than fifty years and some of the original physicians even delivered one of my sisters and my brother. When I called in, they couldn't find me in the new electronic health records system right away. I was talking to a scheduler and she told me that since I hadn't been seen by anyone in the practice for two years, I'd have to be seen as a *new patient* and that they couldn't get me in for at least two weeks because they weren't accepting new patients at that time.

This floored me. I'd just gone through the worst medical crisis of my life and my own doctor's office couldn't see me. I knew I was talking to a scheduler and not to a medical professional and tried to be patient. It wasn't her fault. She was just doing her job. I reiterated my story and added in a bit more detail to try to impress on her a sense of urgency about my situation. I needed to have my stitches taken out and I needed to be examined in the United States for my own peace of mind. I felt both a mixture of frustration and humor that I'd received amazing care—no questions asked—in a foreign country that most Americans would classify as third world; yet the American medical system, held up by many to be the best in the world, wasn't going to give me the time of day.

"Should I go to an urgent care center or the ER to have my stitches removed?" I asked on the phone. "That way, they could refer me to your office for follow-up care."

As I heard myself saying this out loud, I realized the absurdity it. It was the only solution I could think of at the time. There was silence for a split second before the scheduler said, "That seems a little extreme. Let me share this information with the office. Someone will get back with you today."

Later, a nurse called me.

"Mrs. Cross?" she asked. "We've found your file, but since you haven't been seen by anyone for two years, we have to treat you as if you were a new patient."

"I just got back to the States from the Caribbean where I had emergency surgery because my appendix ruptured," I said, pausing to let that sink in. "The doctor there told me that the stiches needed to come out on Tuesday and I'm trying to schedule that follow-up. I also want to be seen by my own doctor to make sure that I'm still recovering from everything okay." I went on to explain my situation in medical terms from the Dominican hospital report. That got her attention.

"Oh my goodness," she exclaimed. "You absolutely do need to be seen. I didn't have all this information before. Let's see what we can do."

At last! The voice of reason! I'm telling you . . . nurses are the unsung heroes of the medical profession.

My first appointment was with a nurse practitioner early the second week home. I was happy to see her, and she proved to be an excellent medical professional. Like most who hear our story, she was horrified. She was also anxious to get my medical info in the system. I'd lost close to thirty pounds by then, but my vitals were within normal ranges. She asked me a lot of questions about my mental state and I was honest with her about what I'd been experiencing. I also told her that I'd had trouble breathing and that it felt like I couldn't draw a complete breath or fully empty my lungs of air when I exhaled. I had Jon stay in the room the whole time because I was still losing my words midsentence and needed his help to tell my story and to remember the details of what she told me.

The NP was incredibly compassionate. She asked me if I felt like I needed anything to ease my anxiety or if I wanted to talk to anyone. I declined and said that I wanted to follow a more natural route for now. She supported that, but she said that I should reach out if I wanted to change anything.

As the NP started to remove my stitches to check the wound further and apply a new bandage, she cut the stitches and then realized that the sutures were partially inside of me and the suture thread needed to be pulled out rather than cut out.

"I'm going to stop right here," she said. "Everything's okay, but you need someone with more experience than I have at removing these kinds of stitches." Jon and I looked at each other as she got one of the doctors in the practice. I had a momentary flash of panic at the idea that we'd come so far only to be tripped up by removal of my stitches in a US medical facility! My fears were unfounded, however: the doctor came in to assist and all was well. The NP wanted me to have some bloodwork done and then said I needed to be off work until mid-March or so—about four weeks—and consider part-time after that until April or May. She also said that I needed to keep walking regularly. At my follow-up appointment, we'd discuss adding any other forms of exercise.

With the stitches out, I was cleared to shower. Yay! I made Jon stay in the house with me until I was done with my first shower in case I fell or passed out. I don't think I've ever enjoyed a shower more. I was still having trouble standing up for long periods of time and in a lot of pain. That said, standing in the warm water was life-giving in its own way. A simple shower. I vowed to appreciate the fact that I was still around to take one. After so many days of bathing with wipes and not being able to wash my hair easily, I felt reborn. It was wonderful to feel clean! I do have to admit that my first shower wiped me out physically. I had to brace myself against the wall while I dried my hair with a blow dryer. I took a long nap afterward.

The kids continued to check in regularly.

Me: Two walks down driveway today. Very slow and had to take naps afterward but I did it! Taking it one day at a time.

Katie: That's a mile! Good job!

Me: Hope you guys are having a good week so far. Doubled my walking again. Up and down the driveway four times (two times twice). Tired, but good to be walking more. Still feeling a little bruised. I'm getting stronger every day! Love you guys. You've been amazing through all of this.

Katie: Good job, mom! I bet it's so nice to get outside and walk around in fresh air

Me: It is. Supposed to be warmer over the weekend too. Yay!

Jimmy: How are you feeling?

Me: My stamina stinks but I'm feeling better every day. Scars have scabs forming and are a little tender but able to move better and bend more.

Jimmy: How are u mentally?

Me: Less nervous than I was but still a little jumpy. A door slammed in the wind yesterday and I nearly jumped out of my shoes. I'm feeling more rested and able to focus for sure, which is good. Still get a little emotional sometimes. Dad and I have been talking a lot and debriefing each other about everything.

I've also been journaling. Definitely not keeping it all in.

Jimmy: Excellent! Glad to hear that progress has been made. The stamina will come. Are u eating ok? or better?

Me: Thanks, Mur. I appreciate your support. You're a good son. It means a lot that you keep checking on me.

Jimmy: The more u exercise and use your muscles at this point the better (without overdoing it of course). Increased blood flow and strength = increased faster healing.

Me: Got it RE exercise. Been increasing my walking every day and also doing some household stuff that makes me stand up for longer periods of time. I take breaks and naps when needed. It's all helping. I think I'm doing pretty well considering it's only been three weeks since the surgery and two since I've been home. Thanks for checking in. Heading out for a walk now. Gorgeous here today — 63!

Jimmy: I think you're doing fantastic. One day at a time, no rush on this

The bloodwork ordered by the NP showed that while my blood sugar was okay, my cholesterol was very high. This surprised me since in the past it had barely registered. The NP said that it wasn't abnormal for my body chemistry to be out of whack after such a trauma. I was eating a very healthy diet and walking as much as I could tolerate every day. She wanted to repeat the same bloodwork in July, near my six-month postsurgery date and she also wanted a colonoscopy to make sure that I had fully healed from the inside. I didn't need to see her until late February, at which time I expected to learn what else I could do exercise-wise.

By this time I was sleeping better but still having trouble relaxing. I knew I was safe. I'd also minimized any noise and distractions. I just couldn't concentrate for any length of time and I'd wake up really early in the morning feeling jumpy and anxious.

One of my nieces, a nurse working third shift, went home in the early morning and would often text me. Those messages were a lifeline for me. Her husband has his private pilot's license and she'd often send me some gorgeous photos to lift my spirits. She was also good to talk with because she suffers from ulcerative colitis and has had some medical battles herself. I shared with her my need to keep my world very small.

> **Niece:** Recovery is the battle! But you're a strong person! I know you will do well.
>
> **Me:** Thanks. Beautiful photo. Keep your texts and photos coming. They help a lot and calm me. This is weird for me. I know how sick you were last year but it's going to take some mental time to work through what I've just experienced. You're the only family member I can think of who's come even close to this.
>
> **Niece:** Well, I was very sick, unable to get better for many months. I had 3 blood transfusion, 1 infusion of iron and didn't eat for over a month. I probably have a really good idea. I would be more than happy to listen, if you wanted to talk about it. Confidentiality intact.
>
> **Me:** And you still live with it. I'll try not to overstay my welcome but thank you for all of your support. I'm on the mend and will be fully recovering. Appreciate everything. Nice to have my own team on standby. Love you. You are one impressive lady.

I added one more layer to my medical team when I went to see my chiropractor in the first few weeks of my recovery. When I turned fifty, I started seeing a chiropractor as part of my ongoing investment in my own health. Jon had been going for a while and I could see the benefits in him. At that time, I was planning to live to be one hundred, so I figured I needed to do anything I could to keep my body shored up. I thought I was feeling good before those very first visits at age fifty, but after being in regular treatment for a few years, I realized that I'd been fooling myself. My body felt so much better! I could move better. My seasonal allergies were easier to manage. And I slept better.

At my first appointment postsurgery, I explained to my doctor what had happened. I also explained that I couldn't handle any adjustments that required me to lie on my stomach because I was still physically unable to do so. In addition, I explained that I had developed bursitis in my right hip. He understood completely and examined me carefully. He then explained what he could do to aid in my healing. The doctor made a few changes to my overall adjustment plan to address the physical issues I'd described and to support the recovery of my immune system, which had been working overtime since my appendix ruptured.

There are many who question the validity of chiropractic medicine. I used to be one of them. Well, I'm a convert for life. The use of the nontraditional healing method mixed in with standard Western medicine was just the boost I needed to keep my recovery on track. I was scheduled to see my chiropractor every week for at least one month, after which we'd reevaluate and decide what was needed next.

My chiropractor also helped to restore some of my faith in US medical professionals. While my medical doctor's office ended up being great to work with and my NP is outstanding (and the professional I ask for by name when I need treatment in their office), the barriers I had to overcome to get in to see them had soured me a little on medical people.

Never once in Dominica did anyone put forward any type of obstacle to treating me. I knew I wasn't a typical Dominican patient. I was a foreigner with no medical history as far as they were concerned. I wasn't their first appendectomy case and I knew I wouldn't be their last, but they treated me as if I were their most important every time they talked to me. Every. Single. Time. No barriers. No protocols. Just an honest-to-goodness desire to help me feel better.

My chiropractor shared that same perspective. He treated me with the same high degree of respect and compassion I'd experienced in Dominica simply because I needed his help. It was humbling.

Letting the World Back In

Icontinued to increase my walking distance and pace. My breathing issues were slowly resolving themselves the more I rested and relaxed in quiet. They seemed to be a byproduct of the environmental factors Dr. Theodore believed and my own body's reaction to the mental issues I experienced. They definitely weren't getting any worse and I never had to contact the NP about them. By the third week postsurgery, I was ready for a few visitors. My mom and one of my sisters were the first to come by. They brought an amazing lunch (with lots of leftovers for Jon and me!) and stayed for a few hours. When they first saw me, they were a little surprised. My hair was a lot longer because I hadn't had it cut for two months and my weight loss was evident. I was also very pale.

We hugged and cried. The hugs were different than the ones we usually exchanged. We're a hugging family and are used to wrapping each other up in love and support when we hug. This time, the hugs—like those from the kids—were full of relief and gratitude in addition to the love. I could really feel that they were transferring to me positive energy and emotion. It was wonderful! Again, like the hugs from the kids, I felt surrounded in white light. I didn't see it emanating from them as I did with the kids, but I could feel its effects just the same.

As my sister was getting lunch out, we sat at the table to talk. My mom was sitting to my left and kept holding my hand or rubbing my arm. I think she was trying to reassure herself that I really was alive and well. I realized in that moment how much what had happened to Jon and to me had impacted so many others. It's not that I'd disregarded this. I just didn't fully understand the extent of it. We had a wonderful visit. Jon stayed close by and filled in some gaps when I couldn't remember parts of our experience. I was absolutely exhausted when they left and had to take a nap. I also had to keep the noise at a minimum to rest my brain. Their visit was the perfect first step in letting the world back in to my life, but I realized that I still had to keep it controlled and small.

That same week, one of my bosses also came to visit and brought some delicious food. Like the others before her, she was visibly affected by what she saw of me. It was again that mix of *she's really alive* and *wow, she looks so different*. I shared my story with her (my first time without help from Jon), including my out-of-body experience, and she was moved. She said she even got goose bumps! I could feel her genuine compassion. It meant so much to me that she'd come by. I knew she'd be reporting back in to the folks at work. They had all been so amazing. Their food, prayers, email, and concern were making a huge difference in my recovery.

I had one other visitor that week. One of my dearest friends of nearly ten years stopped by with a care package full of fun. She brought silly hats, old-fashioned games, and some sleeves that looked like tattoos once you put them on. She also brought a metal watering can that looked like a cheerful bluebird. She'd been texting and emailing me throughout my recovery, but when she saw me for the first time, I could tell that she had the same mixed feelings I'd seen on others of gratitude, relief, compassion, and love.

"I'm so glad to see you," she said as I handed her a mug of hot tea. We sat down for a visit and she immediately started telling me funny stories about her cat, an energetic, gorgeous Maine Coon kitten with a penchant for getting into trouble.

I laughed a lot. It felt so good to laugh again! My mind cleared and I was able to breathe easily. What a gift her visit was. To this day, that bluebird sits on the corner of my kitchen counter as a reminder of the value of true friendship and of humor. In fact, it's almost always something that others who come in my kitchen comment on and admire.

———

At my follow-up appointment in late February, my NP cleared me to go to yoga. I still had some anxious moments and I was forgetting words still, but my breathing was almost back to normal, I was up to four to five miles of walking each day and my stamina was coming back slowly. I realized, though, that I'd lost a lot of mobility, flexibility, and strength. It was time to take baby steps to regain those.

I'd been taking yoga classes on and off for a few years at this great gym in my hometown. The gym owner is a breast cancer survivor and opened her own gym as a way of giving back to the world by helping people to use exercise to help themselves lead healthier lives. She offers a mix of classes for all ages and is a bundle of energy and smarts. Gym members and class participants are like a big family cheering each other on. It's a place of positive energy and white light. Taking any class other than yoga was out of the question until at least April—they were simply too strenuous. Yoga was my only option.

When I decided to try my first class, I arrived early to talk to my instructor. I haven't taken yoga from many different instructors, but I'd bet that she's one of the most nontraditional I've ever met, which in my book makes her one of the best. We have a connection outside of yoga because she and her husband now live in my mother-in-law's old house, one where Jon spent many of his growing-up years. It makes both Jon and me happy that his family home is nurturing another family. In yoga class, she's incredibly focused on making sure that everyone is safe, first and foremost. At the same time, she also makes it fun. She hugs everyone when they come in, shares stories, and makes funny sounds when any of us—including her—tips over during balance moves. She also laughs. A lot. When I work out with her I feel physically stronger, more alert mentally, and as if my spirit has gotten a booster shot.

I met with her and briefly explained what had happened to me because I wanted to reassure her that I'd been cleared to do yoga. (I'd also shared this with the gym owner.) She was so curious about how I was feeling emotionally and how we'd gotten through all of it that during our conversation, I also felt moved to share with her my out-of-body experience. We both cried. By that time others were coming to class and she had to get things started. She offered me options for every move that might put pressure on my atrophied muscles. I could also feel her watching me closely and sending me some of her positive energy.

That first class was hard, and I had to take a nap after I got home, but it was also a turning point in my recovery. My body was starting to smile back at me rather than complain. I knew I'd push through and return to good health in mind, body, and spirit.

Eventually I was cleared to go back to work, add more strenuous workouts to my routine, and resume more of my previous life. However, my mixed-up brain issues lingered until early June. I was back in most ways, but I still ran into times when I had to really concentrate on what I was saying to get all the words out. My brain thought of the words and I was very much present in the conversation, but sometimes between my brain and my mouth, the words got lost. We never identified a specific cause of this other than it was my own way of dealing with what had happened. My brain just needed time to recalibrate itself. I also passed all my follow-up blood tests and my colonoscopy. It was weird to see my scars from the inside, but if they were considered healthy and normal by the doctors, they could look like whatever they needed to as far as I was concerned.

Each time I encountered a friend, family member, or loved one for the first time, their reactions were the same. First, they hugged me as if they had to reassure themselves that I was real. Then, they cried—and I usually did too, as I received their love for me. Then, they'd look at me as if I was different, yet the same, as though I had transcended something that they wanted to be able to understand but might not be able to. I've tried to accept this mix of curiosity and compassion as the love it's intended to be and with grace. Sometimes I do that well. At other times, it's been a little forced. But, in the end, all the time, it's with profound gratitude and humility. I am healthy. I am alive. I matter. I am loved.

Learning to Let My Light Shine Through

The messages of pure love and acceptance I received in my near-death experience came across to me as sacred truths. I was loved. I was enough. I didn't need to hide the real me from the world. I have to admit, though, that it took some time to trust myself to live them. In some ways, I'm still discovering what that means.

As I mentioned at the beginning of this story, I learned at an early age to hide part of my true self from the world in order to fit into it. I believed that me as me simply wasn't good enough. I had to hold back parts of myself that others weren't ready to accept despite circumstances that kept pushing me front and center. I totally missed the fact that this perspective was crushing my spirit in many ways and I was becoming disconnected from myself.

My first two weeks back in the States, where I rested in quiet, enabled my spirit to have some moments of clarity. I realized that I no longer wanted to live a disconnected life. I'd experienced what it felt like for people to accept me as me while I was in Dominica, and although I still felt vulnerable (a lifetime of hiding my light wasn't something I could overcome quickly), I no longer felt the same fear or shame about being myself. This was the beginning of my spiritual recovery.

Since this disruption, people often tell me that they want to be part of my energy or that they like being near me. They tell me I give off a good vibe that makes them feel better somehow. I'm trying hard to embrace and trust the authenticity of their words by being fully present when I'm with others. Interestingly enough, it's brought me back in touch with something that I've let simmer under my surface for many years and I like it. Let me explain.

Since I was a child, people have noticed and remembered me. They often seek me out for no apparent reason. I can be in a crowd of strangers and walk away with new friends and people who remember details about me from the briefest of encounters. A boss I once had referred to it as being confident in my own voice. For me, it's just something that happens. It isn't intentional or planned. It's just me.

When Jon and I are out together, people we meet—even those who are more connected to him than to me—tend to look more at me and speak more directly to me than to him. We've even been places where he's led a conversation, only to have me walk up and the person with whom he's been speaking redirects everything my way—and on subjects that I know nothing about!

I've also been in professional settings supporting a client, a prospect, a boss, or another VIP and received attention inadvertently that should have been directed at the other person. That doesn't always go over well because it has often been misinterpreted as me trying to take center stage. Over the years, I've learned to deflect and redirect this attention back to others and not take so personally the negative remarks that come my way when this happens.

I've never understood this attraction people have to me, to be honest, but have remained curious about it. A few years back, I had my aura read, thinking I might learn more about what makes me, me and why others want to be around me. I believe auras represent energy fields that surround all living beings. The colors that radiate from each being reflect their experiences and feelings. Maybe I could find some answers.

My aura, I learned, was a halo of white, purple, and light fuchsia with touches of blue, colors I saw in my bubble of light in Dominica. According to the guide given to me at the time of the reading, my light combination represents divine energy, spiritual motivation, angels, spirit guides, cosmic wisdom, intense energy, intuition, creative imagination, healing abilities, communication, the desire to help others, unconditional love, and oneness. I'm a seeker of harmony, peace, spiritual growth, and rejuvenation.

After the aura reading, Jon nicknamed me "Violet" as a way of reminding me to be in touch with all that was good about me. He wanted me to trust life and not try to micromanage it so much. For me at that time, his challenge was easier said than done.

My greatest spiritual relearning, after all I've been through, has been how to be present in the moments of my life rather than directing them so much. *Existence living* isn't my calling, even though it had masqueraded as such. What I now know for sure is that I've survived up to this point to be of service to others in an authentic way through presence, brainpower, confidence, positivity, and joy-filling.

With this renewed spirit, I was excited to go back to work. Truth be told, I'd felt restless before my vacation but had convinced myself that the intense pace of the work was getting to me rather than recognizing that the job was no longer the right fit. Before my first official day, Jon and I hosted a small party to thank everyone for their love and support during our time of need. The event was on a Friday afternoon and I was scheduled to go back part-time the following week.

The party was a lot of fun. The whole office was there to celebrate my recovery and hear more about my story. It was relaxing, and Jon and I toasted everyone present. The positive energy of that day lasted just under a month. The work and clients I loved were still the same, but I realized that I'd changed. My passion was no longer enough to overcome the logistics of a traditional schedule, and the politics of the office environment crushed my spirit. I knew I had the power to change things, but as one of the wage-earners in our household, I knew I wouldn't just quit without having some type of plan in mind. What was I going to do? Did I want to go to another agency? Re-enter corporate America? Do something totally different? I just didn't see a clear path forward.

I polished my resumé and started covertly scouting new opportunities. Still, I hesitated to make the leap. My old self-doubts crept back in.

By midsummer, my conflicted feelings and unhappiness were peaking and I was close to a break point. My boss approached me with an opportunity to become a contracted employee rather than a full-time one, and I accepted. I set up shop as a freelance public relations consultant. Jon helped me to create a workspace we affectionately call "The Girl Room" because it is 100 percent me, an eclectic mix of art, traditional office, and unstructured space that feeds my soul. I've steadily grown my client base doing work that I love and am good at and, best of all, I'm making time to live my life rather than checklist it. I feel like my mind, body, and spirit have been realigned.

Afterthoughts — Jon

It's easy now to think back on the sequence of events and realize that everything happened exactly as it needed to and may even have been divinely orchestrated. At every turn, the right next thing happened and the right people were available to help us prepare ahead of our trip and to help get us through everything once the worst started to happen. This includes our kids, who are pretty amazing.

When Susan and I got back from Dominica I wanted to capture all my thoughts and memories about our adventure while they were still fresh in my mind. Most of what I wrote was done within days of our return home. The emotion was still raw. We were both exhausted and Susan was fighting hard to heal physically, emotionally, and spiritually. While she spent a lot of time sleeping, I wrote down my portion of the story. It was important for me to get it out right away. At the time I didn't understand why Susan wasn't doing the same. Now I know that she just wasn't able or ready then.

As I write this now, nearly a year has gone by. A lot has happened since Dominica, but the memories are still vivid. Susan and I talk about what happened and occasionally something new comes up that one or the other didn't know. We have gone about our lives and have been sucked back into the *blackness* of the *real world* a time or two. Funny how we can't seem to resist the pull from what we too often consider to be important, but really isn't. We just do.

The life that Susan and I have together is relatively quiet and calm. We don't do drama very well and we work hard to avoid it. We enjoy an off-the-beaten-path trip now and again, which others have considered adventures. Our adventure in Dominica was certainly tame compared to the stories others in this world have shared, but things like this normally don't happen to us.

Let's face it, from everything we know now, Susan was hours, maybe minutes away from death. She was doing everything physically possible to fight for her life. I was very close to having to figure out how to get her body home from the Caribbean rather than helping her heal so we could come home together. That's a very sobering thought. A thought that forced me to take inventory of what was really important in this life.

We have a little chalkboard that hangs on the wall in our dining room. Usually it has things written on it like dates to remember, groceries to pick up, important phone numbers, and so on. Within the first couple of months after we got home we removed everything on it and added just three things. This is what is says now:

Live Life Fearlessly

Trust Life

FEAR = Face Everything And Rise

It's hard for me to decide what one thing I am most grateful for throughout our adventure. There are just too many good things that have come out of it. Words can't describe our gratitude toward the people in Dominica who helped us so unselfishly. Family and friends have also been incredibly supportive. Everyone has expressed their concern and amazement at the details of our story. All of that support has been very helpful.

As the months have gone by since we got home, I think the one thing that is most important to me is that Susan and I went through this together. Susan is the one who went through the medical emergency in a small foreign country. She was the one who was bathed in light and felt divine presence. Her near-death experience has allowed her to find pieces of her true self that have been covered up for a lot of years, which she so eloquently writes about in this book. And while she experienced all of the medical trauma firsthand, we absolutely went through this together. What I watched her experience has impacted me as much as it has her. What we experienced together in Dominica will always be uniquely ours. Even the details in this book cannot adequately capture the emotion of the adventure.

Susan's body was dying, but even so she was still worried about my well-being. While she fought hard to stay alive, one of her main concerns was still me. She wanted to make sure I was comfortable, had people to watch after me, and that I was okay. This was all while she was stuck in pretty miserable conditions that she couldn't control. She has always been my biggest cheerleader throughout our marriage, but I don't know that I fully understood her love for me and my spirit until this happened.

Susan said that while she was healing in the hospital she couldn't pray for herself, something that has never happened to her before. However, she was still able to easily pray for others. She could pray for me. She could pray for all the other women in the ward with her who were in as much pain as she was. She could give love to others around her even during a time of personal desperation. I saw how miserable she was for nearly a week. I watched her clinging to life, and I also watched her give her love to others unselfishly. What an amazing thing to witness!

It was OUR adventure together. It wasn't one we expected or signed up for, but one that we have both grown from individually and as a couple. It was what we both needed to have happen to us. We are richer from the experience and try to approach life in a different way now. Isn't that what we're all here for? Learn from the good and the bad, and through all of it experience love in the not-so-obvious places.

Life can change in an instant. We found that out on our trip. The people of Dominica also found that out in September of 2017 when Hurricane Maria made a direct hit on the tiny island. According to news reports and pictures, the island was devastated. We were heartbroken to think about our friends who helped us while we were there.

Not long after the hurricane I emailed Hervé to see if he was okay. He responded quickly. He remembered us and was glad to know Susan was doing well. He said the island was stripped bare of vegetation and all buildings were damaged. However, he said nature will grow back and nothing was beyond repair. He had posts on his Facebook page of his involvement with flying to nearby islands to pick up supplies for his fellow Dominicans.

Only about seventy-five thousand people live in Dominica. More people will watch a college football game in any given stadium on a fall Saturday in the United States. It's a small country on a small island, but they take care of each other. They took care of us. It's what they do.

Afterthoughts — Susan

I think that many people expect someone who goes through something like I did to have some profound learning or life-altering change of course. That's too dramatic for me. I've definitely had a shift in how I approach the world, but as I've said, I think it's more of a reconnect with part of my soul that I'd let linger in the background for too long. We've been taught to fear life disruptions, but this disruption has caused an eruption in me in the best way possible. It cleared a lot of life debris for me. I am different. I'm also the same. Most importantly, I'm giving myself permission to live more of my authentic life rather than existing in a life dictated by circumstances or by others.

My life before my appendix ruptured was such a whirlwind of activity while I tried to prove my worth, that I can see now that I wasn't always nurturing my true self. Don't get me wrong, I experienced a lot of happiness, but I didn't always give myself permission to convey that childlike sense of wonder and joy that feeds the spirit.

I had very high control needs about the world around me. When there's a problem, that perspective is well received because people generally want someone to be in charge and to fix whatever's going wrong. That expectation was one I felt often. When life was going along at its own pace, well, let's just say that I could come across as domineering and brittle.

My experiences in Dominica and after I returned home were a major wake-up call for me. Although I might have appreciated a little less drama as the universe was trying to get my attention, I'd gone so far off track that I'm not sure I could have found my way through on my own. Also, if anything had happened any differently, I don't think I'd feel so renewed. It took close to a year for me to see this and I'm still learning. I hope I never stop. I'm perpetually recovering my own sense of fun. I find joy in the simplest things. My brain is cranking out ideas like it used to do way back when I gave it the space and grace to think. I feel so much life every single day.

I believe that my out-of-body experience set the stage for my transformation. First, I needed to be reassured that I was enough. Period. I didn't need to achieve anything. I didn't need to be someone else or do something differently. I just needed to be me—the heart and soul of my own story. While my main takeaway at the time was that I wasn't going to die, I've come to appreciate that if I hadn't been reassured that I had so much value as a spiritual being (as we all do), I might not have been able to give and receive the pure love that I needed to heal. I might have physically recovered, but I'd still have a broken or wounded spirit. From my vantage point, a broken or wounded spirit that is unable to surrender and be held by others is a spirit that is dying.

I believe that the blackness that I experienced was a symbol of my broken spirit. It represented a false path to *repair* my spirit, but not to restore it. At times, it felt like I needed every weapon in my personal arsenal to stay far back from the blackness void. The traits that I've been chastised personally and professionally for—boldness, strength, confidence, fortitude, intelligence, bossiness, force of will, presence, focus—and those traits I don't always receive credit for—faith, forgiveness, love, acceptance, humility, nurture, humor, compassion, generosity—united to serve me well. I said no over and over and over again when presented with the choice of staying true to my course or surrendering to the easier path of blackness.

As Jon and all the others who were helping us and praying for me showed me, I didn't need to have all the answers. I simply needed to stop holding on and allow myself to be held spiritually in their divine light and physically in their arms. This wasn't a one-time offer. I don't need to hold it together. I need to accept and share love with as many people as I can, every chance that I can.

Second, I needed to rejoin my life. As I realized many times along my health journey, I'd allowed the situations of my life to dictate the circumstances of my life. What do I mean by that? For starters, I worked a lot. I love working because it's challenging and it gives my brain an outlet for all the things that I'm thinking about. It also surrounds me with smart, funny, and creative people. I've been fortunate to do a lot of really amazing things.

As much as I've loved what I was doing and many of the people I've worked with, I can see now that I was taking it way too seriously. I put too much emphasis on the achievement of work—all work, not just my contributions to it—rather than the simpler joy of bringing ideas to life. I was on the brink of living to work rather than working to live. I checked in on vacation. I was almost always tethered to technology. I have a two-year medical history gap because I *forgot* to make time for self-care. I could check off a long list of professional accomplishments (which many others have contributed to and which I am proud of), but I was fitting in my life list. That's just not the way to live.

Third, I needed to express my true appreciation for the authentic spirits of my tribe, starting with my kids and husband. I've always tried to be there for them. I always try to think of them first. I also tell them every chance I get how much I love them and am proud of them. I have also tried to sway them to my way of thinking a time or two when I should have been paying attention to what they were really saying or sharing.

The simple fact is that Jon and I raised two great kids. We didn't do that on our own. Katie and Jimmy are the sum of all the experiences they've had and all the people they've met along the way. Many of those have nothing to do with us. Katie and Jimmy are smart, amazing adults who are a source of light and joy to so many others. Their souls are intact and as they become more confident in the source of their own authentic power, they will continue to have great-filled lives. They each have more strength in them than they realize. If I had died, I know that they would have been okay; but I'm grateful that I'm going to be around to watch their lights grow into full-fledged flames.

As for Jon . . . I married the right man for me. We sometimes laugh and say that we've grown up together and, in many ways, I think we have. When we embarked on our shared journey, neither one of us had any idea how it would turn out. I'm glad we didn't because it's been so much harder and so much richer than anything we could have ever imagined. We might have been scared off if we had known what was in store for us, and then we'd have missed out on so much.

If Dominica taught me anything, it's that Jon and I are soul mates. He's hung in there with me through a lot and balanced me when I didn't even realize it. We don't always agree—and I hope that we never do—but that's what makes it so worthwhile. We see each other through the lens of pure love. We're not trying to change each other. We just want to be present with each other and those in our lives in every moment.

As for the rest of my tribe, which is made of loved ones I know and friends I have yet to meet, I honor you. I respect you and I hope that my presence in your life can be as much of a gift to you as yours is to me.

My hope is that each of us will choose to fill our lives with wonder and joy. It's the only way we can navigate life's disruptions.

How?

Trust your tribe. We each have a tribe of family and loved ones. We also have a much wider circle made up of people who show up unannounced just because we need them. We may never know all of their names, but they're there and they want to help.

Surrender to silence. Sometimes the boldest, most powerful thing we can do is relax in quiet. It used to be nearly impossible for me. I learned, however, that it's restorative, gives us a chance to reconnect with ourselves, and empowers us to participate in our own life rather than just living it as a checklist.

Live in the now. I was conditioned to think my life should revolve around great moments, but I've come to appreciate that great moments often catch us unaware. They're sometimes beautifully wrapped up in what others would call small moments, and if we're not paying attention we'll miss them. When I see myself as already living my greatest story, I have the patience to ride out disruptive storms, seeing and accepting the gifts being offered up to me along the way.

Let the universe have your back. It sure didn't feel like it at the time, but I've come to see that this storm was part of a clean-up taking place in my life. Blackness doesn't have to win. I'm living proof that my disruption wasn't an end, it's been a beginning.

Believe in yourself enough to go for your joy. I can choose to be a person seeking success or a person of value. I have value just as I am and that's the secret to my success. I need to trust in that and live it.

My story today? Well, let's just say that it's filled with life, love, challenge, anxiety, and beauty. It's also filled with wonder and joy. And I intend to keep it that way. Some of my life's best stories haven't even begun.

Acknowledgments

This book has been one of the hardest and easiest things I've ever done. It was hard because I wanted to be sure I told the story in a way that honors all who lived it directly or indirectly. Getting the details down just right has taken incredible focus and fortitude. It was easy because as I think about what happened to me, I smile. I remain humbled by the love and support I received just because I needed it.

A book is never published in isolation. Although I'm sure I'll forget someone, I'd like to especially thank the following people:

- My husband, Jon, for being my best friend and the love of my life. He is a constant source of encouragement to me and knows just when to bring a little humor into the mix to keep life interesting.

- My daughter, Katie, and son, Jimmy, whose big hearts, big brains, and sense of fun never cease to amaze me.

- My son-in-law, Mike, and daughter-in-law, Megan, for loving my kids unconditionally.

- My large, noisy, silly, extended family. You are the most loving, positive, and joyful people I know.

- ♦ My inner circle of friends who served as readers and editors along the way and who are always cheering me on no matter what I do.

- ♦ Katherine Pickett and Christy Collins for their exceptional editing and design skills. These pros have made this writer look good.

- ♦ The team at Bradley Communications for guiding me in all things publishing and holding me to the highest standards possible. Your counsel has been invaluable.

Thank you. Two simple words with so much meaning. Your presence with me is a gift I treasure.

Contact Susan

To learn more about navigating disruption and creating personal eruptions of the best kind or for information about booking Susan as a speaker, visit: *Susan-Cross.com.*
You can also connect with Susan here:

Blog: susan-cross.com/blog
Facebook: facebook.com/SusanCrossWriter
Instagram: instagram.com/susan_cross_writer

www.ingramcontent.com/pod-product-compliance
Lightning Source LLC
Chambersburg PA
CBHW070927030426
42336CB00014BA/2567